LA

Cooking Without the 8 Major Food Allergens, Plus Corn, Gluten and MSG

Allergy Safe Cuisine

Cooking Without the 8 Major Food Allergens, Plus Corn, Gluten and MSG

FIRST EDITION

This book is dedicated to two special little girls.
Nana loves you!

Please be advised that I am not a medical professional and nothing printed here is intended as medical advice. Always check ingredients before you buy and check them every time, as each person's needs are different and manufacturers may change ingredients at any time. Always seek the advice of your doctor with questions regarding ingredients and food allergies.

ISBN 978-0-615-64633-6
Library of Congress Control Number: 2012909466
Published by JD Incorporated
Printed in the United States of America

Introduction

Living with multiple food allergies does not mean meals have to be bland and flavorless. With Allergy Safe Cuisine, you can create a variety of dishes that are not only distinctive, but delicious as well.

To help you achieve that goal, *Allergy Safe Cuisine* provides 200 recipes to get you started, each one free of the eight major food allergens, plus corn, gluten and MSG. Discover how to transform formerly forbidden recipes into safe and delicious meals, from Chicken Curry Salad and Corned Beef Hash to Cream of Mushroom Soup.

You'll discover a rich variety of side dishes, too. Indulgences such as Spinach, Fennel and Sausage Stuffing and Carrot Ginger Bisque are sure to please when combined with unique ingredients and delicious seasonings and sauces that you can make yourself.

Find out the secrets of creating substitutes for many kitchen staples, such as Worcestershire sauce and sweet pickle relish, with easy to follow recipes and step by step instructions.

You will find that fewer foods than you thought are off limits. There are mouthwatering dips, fresh chutneys and fabulous desserts such as Cilantro-Lime Pesto, Black Bean Dip and Lime Parfait, as well as tasty breakfast foods like Muesli, Banana Donuts and homemade Granola Bars.

In addition to providing you with a great variety of recipes to choose from, this book serves as a basic guide to help create your own special dishes. With a little bit of fun and experimentation, "Allergy Safe Cuisine" will be sure to become an important part of your kitchen in no time!

Table of Contents

Hidden Ingredients

Canned fruits, jams, jellies and fruit juices often contain high fructose corn syrup and ascorbic acid. Ascorbic acid is a synthetic form of Vitamin C, and is derived from corn. Dried fruits may be dusted with corn products to prevent sticking, and are often sweetened to improve taste.

Meats are often brined, soaked or injected with emulsifiers or other ingredients to tenderize, preserve and add flavor. These ingredients can cover all 8 major food allergens, in addition to corn, gluten and MSG. Be especially wary of deli meats, and don't buy meats that share the same counters and equipment as the cheese department.

There are several canned tomato products mentioned in this cookbook, and a check of all the local supermarkets revealed they are readily available. Just read the labels carefully when buying. I did, however, include recipes for tomato sauce and stewed tomatoes on the chance your local supermarket doesn't carry any allergen-free brands.

Some brands of rice milk may contain soy, vanilla, xanthan gum or natural flavorings. The vanilla, xanthan gum and natural flavorings may be derived from corn, so always check with the manufacturer before using if corn is an issue.

Baking products such as flour, sugar, molasses, honey, baking powder and yeast may contain hidden food allergens. I have included safe replacement suggestions or product recommendations for each one of these, with a special section in the back with the actual ingredients and toll-free numbers so you can follow-up again yourself before buying.

Beans and Lentils

Black Bean Chili ~ 7
Boston Baked Beans ~ 8
Cauliflower Chickpea Curry ~ 9
Chickpea Casserole ~ 10
Chick Peas and Cabbage ~ 11
Chile con Carne ~ 12
Curried Lentils ~ 13
Indian Style Lentils ~ 14
Lentil Stuffed Peppers ~ 15
Quinoa Tabouleh ~ 16
Red Beans and Rice ~ 17
Spinach and Bean Dumplings ~ 18

Black Bean Chili

1 medium onion, chopped
1 medium green pepper, chopped small pieces
1 tablespoon extra-virgin olive oil
1-1/2 cups vegetable stock (see recipe)
6 cloves garlic, minced
2 (15-ounce) cans black beans, drained
1 (8-ounce) can tomato sauce (or see recipe)
1 (14-1/2 ounce) can stewed tomatoes, with juice (or see recipe)
2 tablespoons ground cumin
2 tablespoons chili powder
2 tablespoons dried oregano
2 tablespoons jalapenos, sliced
1/4 cup fresh cilantro, chopped
Sea salt and freshly ground black pepper

Heat 1 tablespoon oil in a medium saucepan. Sauté onion and pepper in oil over medium heat about 5 minutes, stirring frequently, until translucent. Add garlic, cumin and red chili powder and continue to sauté another minute. Add stock and rest of ingredients except for cilantro. Simmer 30 more minutes, uncovered. Add cilantro. Season with salt and pepper to taste. Makes 4 servings.

Boston Baked Beans

1-1/2 pound package dried navy beans
1/4 pound additive-free bacon, cooked and crumbled
1 medium onion, sliced into chunks
2 medium onions, peeled and left whole
3/4 cup pure cane dark brown sugar (see note)
1/3 cup corn-free molasses (see note)
2 teaspoons dry mustard
1/2 teaspoon sea salt
1/4 teaspoon freshly ground black pepper
2 cups water

Place dried beans in a large saucepan with enough cold water to cover. Bring to boil over high heat, uncovered. Boil 2 minutes, then remove from heat and set aside for 1 hour. Drain and rinse beans, then return to saucepan. Slice 1 onion into big chunks and to beans. Cover with cold water and bring to boil over high heat. Reduce heat to low and cook beans until tender, about 1-1/2 hours. Drain beans and discard onion. Preheat oven to 350°F. Place remaining 2 onions in large casserole dish or bean pot. Add drained beans and cooked bacon. In small bowl, place sugar, molasses, dry mustard, salt and pepper. Mix well. Stir in water until combined and then pour over beans. Cover casserole dish or bean pot and bake 1-1/2 hours. Uncover and cook another 1/2 hour or so, until beans are tender. Makes 8 servings.

Dark brown sugar can be replaced with 1/2 cup white sugar and 2 tablespoons corn-free molasses or Yacon syrup for each 1/2 cup. Molasses can be replaced with equal amounts Yacon syrup.

Cauliflower Chickpea Curry

1 tablespoon extra-virgin olive oil
1/2 yellow onion, minced
2 cloves garlic
1 teaspoon ginger, minced
1/2 teaspoon cumin
1/2 teaspoon coriander
1 teaspoon turmeric
1/2 teaspoon salt
1/4 teaspoon cayenne pepper
5 cups cauliflower (about 1/2 large head)
1 (25-ounce) can chickpeas, drained and rinsed
1/2 cup water

Heat oil in large skillet. Add onion and sauté until soft, about five minutes. Add garlic and continue to sauté another minute. Add spices, stir and sauté an additional minute. Add chickpeas, cauliflower and water. Stir to mix with sauce. Cover and bring to boil. Turn heat down and simmer 10 minutes, or until cauliflower is tender. Serve over brown basmati rice. Makes 4 to 6 servings.

Chickpea Casserole

1 tablespoon extra-virgin olive oil
2 large onions, thinly sliced
4 garlic cloves, minced
2 small green chilies, seeded and thinly sliced
1 teaspoon ground coriander
1 teaspoon ground cumin
1 teaspoon Garam Masala (see recipe)
1 teaspoon ground turmeric
3 large vine-ripened tomatoes, coarsely chopped
1 teaspoon pure cane light brown sugar
2 tablespoons fresh cilantro or parsley, chopped
2 tablespoons fresh mint, shredded
1/2 cup cooked chickpeas
1 large ripe mango, peeled and cubed

Heat oil in large skillet over medium heat. Add onions and sauté until soft, about 3 to 5 minutes. Add garlic, chilies, coriander, cumin, Garam Masala and turmeric. Reduce heat to medium-low and sauté, stirring constantly, about 2 minutes. Add tomatoes, sugar, half the cilantro and mint, and stir well. Reduce heat to low and simmer about 10 minutes, stirring occasionally, until tomatoes are soft. Stir in chickpeas, cover and simmer about 8 minutes, or until heated through. Stir in mango and simmer until heated through. Pour mixture into warm serving bowl and sprinkle with remaining cilantro and mint. Serve immediately. Makes 4 servings.

Chickpeas and Cabbage

2 tablespoons extra-virgin olive oil
1/2 medium head cabbage, slice thin, then chop into 3-inch segments
1/2 medium onion, sliced thinly
1 carrot, thinly sliced into rounds
3 cloves garlic, minced
1 (15-ounce) can chickpeas, drained and rinsed
1 (14-1/2-ounce) can stewed tomatoes, with juice (or see recipe)
1 teaspoons dried oregano
3 tablespoons fresh parsley, finely chopped
2 tablespoons fresh mint, finely chopped

Heat oil in over medium heat in large skillet. Add onion, cabbage and carrots, cover and cook until mixture begins to brown. Add garlic and stir. Cook for an additional minute. Add chickpeas, stewed tomatoes and oregano. Cover, reduce heat to medium-low, and simmer until cabbage is tender, about 15 minutes. Stir in fresh herbs, cover pan, and cook 5 more minutes. Serve over rice. Makes 4 to 6 servings.

For more of a Moroccan style flavor, you can skip the tomatoes, oregano, parsley and mint, and add 1/2 tablespoon turmeric, 1/2 tablespoon cinnamon, 2 tablespoons corn-free honey, and either 1/4 cup dried currants (for a tart taste), or 1/4 cup raisins (for sweet taste). Add cayenne pepper to taste. These would be added after the mixture begins to brown.

Always use caution when buying honey. Unless you buy certified 100% pure organic, it may contain unlabeled high fructose corn syrup. Honey can be replaced with agave nectar in many recipes.

Chili con Carne

1 tablespoon extra-virgin olive oil
1 large onion, finely chopped
1 medium green Bell pepper, seeded and finely chopped
2 stalks celery, finely chopped
2 to 4 teaspoons chili powder
1 pound organic ground beef, coarsely ground
2 (14-1/2-ounce) cans stewed tomatoes, with juice (or see recipe)
1 (10-ounce) can red kidney beans, drained but not rinsed
1/2 cup water or vegetable stock (see recipe)
Pinch of sea salt

Heat oil in large skillet over medium heat. Add onion and sauté, stirring frequently, until slightly softened, about 3 minutes. Add Bell pepper, celery and chili powder. Cook, stirring frequently, until pepper is slightly tender, about 5 minutes. Transfer vegetables to plate. Increase heat to medium-high and add beef to skillet. Cook, stirring constantly until browned, about 5 minutes. Drain fat and discard. Return vegetables to skillet. Add tomatoes, kidney beans, water and salt. Bring to boil over medium heat, stirring constantly. Reduce heat and simmer, partially covered, stirring occasionally, until beef is tender, about 1 hour. Transfer mixture to serving bowl or plates and serve at once. Makes 4 servings.

Curried Lentils

1 cup lentils, washed
1 tablespoon extra-virgin olive oil
4 cups vegetable stock (see recipe)
1 medium onion, chopped
3 cloves garlic, minced
2 carrots, sliced into 1/4-inch pieces
2 stalks celery, sliced into 1/4-inch pieces
2 cups kale, finely chopped
2 teaspoons curry powder
1 (14-1/2-ounce) can stewed tomatoes, with juice (or see recipe)
3 tablespoons fresh cilantro, chopped
Salt and freshly ground black pepper to taste

Rinse lentils in strainer and let drain. Chop onions and garlic. Heat
1 tablespoon oil over medium heat in a medium sized saucepan.
Sauté onion 5 minutes, until translucent. Add garlic, carrots, and
celery. Sauté few more minutes. Add curry powder and mix. Add
lentils, stock and stewed tomatoes. Bring to boil, reduce heat to
medium-low, and simmer, uncovered, until lentils and vegetables
are tender, about 10 minutes. Add kale and simmer another 10
minutes. Add cilantro and season with salt and freshly ground black
pepper to taste. Makes 4 servings.

Indian Style Lentils

1 medium onion, diced
1 tablespoon extra-virgin olive oil
2 cloves garlic, minced
1 teaspoon dried ginger
1/2 teaspoon turmeric
1/2 teaspoon sea salt
1 cup stewed tomatoes, with juice (see recipe)
2 cups canned or home-cooked lentils
1 cup frozen spinach

Sauté onion in 1 tablespoon oil 3 minutes. Add garlic, ginger, turmeric, salt, stewed tomatoes and lentils. Simmer, covered, approximately 5 to 7 minutes. Add 1 cup frozen spinach and continue simmering 2 more minutes. Serve over brown rice. Makes 4 to 6 servings.

Lentil Stuffed Peppers

2/3 cup red split lentils
4 tablespoons extra-virgin olive oil
4 medium green or red Bell peppers, tops removed and seeded
1 teaspoon cumin seeds
2 onions, finely chopped
2 green chilies, seeded and chopped
1 (1-inch) piece fresh ginger, grated
1 tablespoon ground coriander
1-1/4 cups water
Sea salt and freshly ground pepper to taste
2 tablespoons cilantro, chopped
Cilantro leaves to garnish

Rinse lentils and soak in cold water 30 minutes. Heat half the oil in large skillet over medium-high heat. Add peppers and cook 3 to 5 minutes, until golden brown. Drain on paper towels and let cool. Add remaining oil to skillet. Add cumin seeds and cook until they begin to pop. Add onions and chilies and cook, stirring frequently until onions are soft and golden brown, about 8 minutes. Stir in ginger and cilantro. Drain lentils and add to skillet with 1-1/4 cups of water. Stir well and cover. Reduce heat to low and cook 15 to 20 minutes, until lentils are tender and liquid has evaporated. Stir in salt, pepper and cilantro. Preheat oven to 350°F. Stuff peppers with lentil mixture. Stand in a baking dish. Bake 15 to 20 minutes, until peppers are soft. Serve hot, garnished with cilantro leaves. Makes 4 servings.

Quinoa Tabouleh

1 cup quinoa, rinsed
2 cups water
1 cup Italian parsley, finely chopped
1/2 cup mint leaves, finely chopped
1 cup tomatoes, seeded and chopped
1/2 cup chopped red onion
3 cloves garlic, minced
Juice of 1 lemon
1/3 cup extra-virgin olive oil
Sea salt to taste

Bring water to boil in medium saucepan. Add quinoa, cover, and return to boil. Reduce heat to medium-low and simmer 15 minutes. Remove from heat and let stand 10 minutes, then remove lid and stir. Set aside to cool. Stir in tomatoes, onion and parsley into quinoa. In a small bowl, whisk together lemon juice, oil, garlic and salt. Pour over quinoa mixture and toss well. Cover and refrigerate at least 1 hour before serving. Makes 4 servings.

Red Beans and Rice

1 tablespoon extra-virgin olive oil
1 medium yellow onion, chopped
2 cloves garlic, minced
2 cups peeled diced pumpkin
1/2 teaspoon cumin
1/2 teaspoon turmeric
1/2 teaspoon coriander
1/2 teaspoon cayenne pepper
1/2 teaspoon dried ginger
1 teaspoon sea salt
3 cups water
1-1/2 cups brown basmati rice
1 cup chopped chard
1 (14-ounce) can red kidney beans, drained and rinsed

Heat oil in a large saucepan over medium heat. Add onion and
sauté until tender, about 5 minutes. Add garlic and continue to
sauté for another minute. Stir in rice and spices and cook another
minute. Add water and pumpkin. Stir and bring to boil over
medium-high heat. Reduce heat to medium-low, cover, and simmer
25 minutes. Add beans and chard. Stir, and continue to cook until
all liquid is absorbed and rice is tender, about 15 more minutes.
Remove from heat, fluff rice, and let stand 10 minutes before
serving. Makes 6 servings.

Spinach and Bean Dumplings

1 cup yellow split mung beans
2 ounces frozen spinach, thawed, drained and chopped
2 tablespoons fresh cilantro, chopped
2 green chilies, seeded and chopped
1/4 teaspoon cream of tartar
1/8 teaspoon baking soda
1/2 teaspoon sea salt
Extra-virgin olive oil for deep frying

Put beans in bowl, cover with water and let soak 4 hours. Drain and rinse. Put beans in blender or food processor and process until smooth. Stir in cilantro, chiles, cream of tartar, baking soda and salt. Half-fill a heavy deep skillet or fryer with oil and heat to 375°F, or until a 1-inch bread cube browns in 1 minute. Using a tablespoon, drop mixture into hot oil. Fry 4 to 5 minutes, or until golden brown. Drain dumplings on paper towel and keep warm while cooking remaining mixture. Serve hot. Makes 4 servings.

Beef and Veal

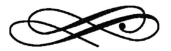

Beef Stew ~ 20
Corned Beef Hash ~ 21
Homemade Beef Jerky ~ 22
Homemade Corned Beef Brisket ~ 23
Liver and Onions ~ 24
Marinated Flank Steak ~ 25
Meatloaf ~ 26
New England Boiled Dinner ~ 27
Shepherd's Pie ~ 28
Stuffed Cabbage Rolls ~ 29
Tropical Spiced Steak ~ 30
Veal Marsala ~ 31
Yankee Pot Roast and Vegetables ~ 32

Beef Stew

2 pounds additive-free beef stew meat, cubed
3 tablespoons extra-virgin olive oil
4 medium carrots, sliced in 1-inch pieces
2 small onions, chopped
1 clove garlic, minced
2 cups red wine
2 cups beef stock (see recipe)
1/4 cup Worcestershire sauce substitute (optional, see recipe)
1 (14-1/2-ounce) can stewed tomatoes, with juice (or see recipe)
1 teaspoon sea salt
1/2 teaspoon dried rosemary
1/2 teaspoon dried thyme
2 bay leaves
8 small red or fingerling potatoes, skin on
1 medium leek, cut into thick rounds
1/2 cup white bean flour for thickener (optional)

Heat 1 tablespoon oil in large skillet over medium-high heat until it begins to smoke. Working in batches, add beef and cook until browned outside. Add more oil if needed. Transfer to large saucepan. Add carrots and onions. When almost browned, add garlic, and sauté until fragrant. Transfer to saucepan. Add a little bit of wine or beef stock to skillet, and stir with wooden spoon to deglaze. Add deglazed mixture to saucepan. Add wine, beef stock, Worcestershire sauce substitute (if using), stewed tomatoes, salt, rosemary, thyme and bay leaves to saucepan and stir. Bring to boil, reduce heat to barely a simmer, partially cover, and cook 1 hour. Add potatoes and leeks and stir. Bring to a boil, reduce heat, and simmer 1 more hour, partially covered. The stew will thicken and intensify in flavor as the liquid evaporates. If thicker stew is desired, whisk 1/2 cup white bean flour with equal amount cold water. Pour into stew slowly, and a little at a time, stirring constantly, until you reach your desired consistency, about 3 to 5 minutes. Remove bay leaves and serve hot. Makes 8 servings.

Corned Beef Hash

2 tablespoons extra-virgin olive oil
1 small onion, finely diced
1 pound homemade corned beef brisket, finely diced (see recipe)
5 small red or yellow potatoes, peeled
1/2 cup beef stock (see recipe)
1 teaspoon prepared yellow mustard
1 teaspoon Worcestershire sauce substitute (optional, see recipe)
Pinch of pure cane sugar
Sea salt and freshly ground black pepper to taste

Boil potatoes in medium saucepan until cooked but still firm. Set aside to cool, then then finely dice. Heat oil in large skillet over medium-high heat. Sauté onions until tender. Add potatoes, corned beef, stock, mustard, Worcestershire sauce substitute and sugar. Add salt and pepper to taste and stir well. Reduce heat, cover and cook 5 minutes. Uncover, stir, cover again, and cook another 5 minutes. Raise heat to medium and cook uncovered until liquid is gone, stirring occasionally. Raise heat to medium-high and cook until hash becomes crusty. Stir, let hash sit for a while and stir again. Serve hot. Makes 4 servings.

Homemade Beef Jerky

2 pounds additive-free lean beef round steak
1/2 cup Coconut Aminos (see note)
1/2 cup water
1 tablespoon white wine vinegar
1 tablespoon pure cane light brown sugar
1 teaspoon fresh ginger, grated
1/4 teaspoon garlic powder
1/4 teaspoon onion powder
1/4 teaspoon cayenne pepper

Trim and discard fat from meat. Cut into long, thin strips 1/4-inch thick. It helps to partially freeze meat for about 45 minutes beforehand. Place in large sealable plastic bag. In medium bowl, combine remaining ingredients. Stir well. Pour over meat and seal. Shake to make sure beef has been evenly coated. Place in refrigerator 24 hours, turning several times. After 24 hours, place wire racks on foil-lined baking sheets. Drain and discard marinade. Place meat strips 1/4-inch apart on racks. Bake uncovered with door propped slightly open, about 1-inch or so, at 160° F for 8 to 10 hours or until meat is dry and leathery. Remove from oven and cool completely. Refrigerate or freeze in an airtight container. Makes 2 pounds beef jerky.

Coconut Aminos can be substituted for soy sauce in dressings, marinades and other recipes. This product is not derived from the nut of the coconut tree.

Homemade Corned Beef Brisket

1 (4 to 5 pound) additive-free beef brisket, trimmed
2 quarts water
1 cup kosher salt
1/2 cup pure cane light brown sugar
1 (3-inch) cinnamon stick, broken into several pieces
1 teaspoon mustard seeds
1 teaspoon black peppercorns
8 whole cloves
8 whole allspice berries
12 whole juniper berries
2 bay leaves, crumbled
1/2 teaspoon dried ginger

Place water in large saucepan along with salt, sugar, cinnamon stick, mustard seeds, peppercorns, cloves, allspice, juniper berries, bay leaves and ginger. Cook over high heat until salt and sugar has dissolved. Remove brine from heat and cool. Refrigerate until it reaches 45°F. Once brine has cooled, place brisket in sealable bag or container and add brine. Seal and place in refrigerator for at least 10 days. Flip brisket over daily, making sure brisket is completely submerged each time. After 10 days, rinse under cold water, and cook according to your favorite recipe.

Cooking the Beef Brisket

1 small onion, quartered
1 large carrot, coarsely chopped
1 stalk celery, coarsely chopped
1 homemade corned beef brisket

Place brisket in saucepan just large enough to hold meat. Add onion, carrot and celery, and cover with water. Bring to boil, reduce heat to low, cover and simmer gently 3 hours or until the meat is fork tender. Remove from pot and slice thinly across grain.

This brisket can also be used in New England Boiled Dinner and Corned Beef Hash. See recipes in the Beef and Veal section.

Liver and Onions

1 pound calf's liver
1/4 cup sunflower seeds, ground
1/4 teaspoon sea salt
1/4 teaspoon black pepper
1 teaspoon dried sage

Topping:
2 medium onions, cut in half and sliced thin
3 medium cloves garlic, minced
2 tablespoons balsamic vinegar
1/2 cup chicken stock (see recipe)
1 tablespoon extra-virgin olive oil
2 tablespoon fresh thyme, chopped
Sea salt and freshly ground black pepper to taste

Turn broiler on high and place a metal oven-proof pan about 7-inches underneath heat source. Heat pan for about 10 minutes. While pan is getting hot, heat oil in large skillet over medium-high heat. Sauté onions 15 minutes, stirring frequently. Add garlic, thyme and vinegar. Mix and add stock. Continue to cook another couple of minutes. While onions are cooking, mix ground sunflower seeds with sage, salt and pepper. Dust liver with mixture. Remove hot pan from broiler and place liver on it. Return to oven, reduce heat to low, and broil about 3 to 5 minutes depending on thickness of liver. Do not turn, as it is cooking on both sides simultaneously. Serve topped with onions. Makes 4 servings.

Marinated Flank Steak

1 additive-free flank steak (about 1-1/2 pounds)
1/2 cup Coconut Aminos (see note)
1/2 cup cream sherry
2 tablespoons extra-virgin olive oil
2 cloves garlic, minced
2 teaspoons fresh ginger, grated
1/4 teaspoon cayenne pepper

Place steak in large sealable plastic bag. In medium bowl, combine rest of ingredients and mix well. Pour over meat and seal. Turn to make sure steak has been evenly coated. Refrigerate 8 hours or overnight, turning occasionally. Drain and discard marinade. Grill, covered, over medium-high heat 6 to 10 minutes on each side, or until meat reaches desired tenderness. For rare, a meat thermometer should read 140° F, medium 160° F, and well-done 170° F. Makes 4 to 6 servings.

Coconut Aminos can be substituted for soy sauce in dressings, marinades and other recipes. This product is not derived from the nut of the coconut tree.

Meatloaf

1-1/2 pounds additive-free ground beef
1/3 cup additive-free ketchup plus 1/3 cup for top (see recipe)
1/3 cup Worchester sauce substitute (see recipe)
1/2 teaspoon celery salt
1 teaspoon garlic powder
1 onion, chopped
Sea salt and freshly ground pepper to taste
3 slices (roughly 1 cup) bread, toasted, torn into small pieces (see
    recipe)
2 tablespoons pure cane light brown sugar
2 tablespoons prepared yellow mustard

Preheat oven to 350° F. In large bowl, combine ground beef, 1/3 cup ketchup, Worchester sauce substitute, celery salt, garlic powder, salt and pepper, and squish together with clean hands. Add onion and bread and work into mixture. Shape into loaf and place on lightly greased baking dish. In small bowl, combine 1/3 cup ketchup, brown sugar and mustard. Coat top of meatloaf with thick layer of mixture. Cook 1 hour, or until done. If meatloaf starts to brown too much, cover loosely with foil tent during last 15 minutes or so. Makes 8 servings.

New England Boiled Dinner

4 pounds homemade corned beef brisket (see recipe)
6 to 8 carrots, peeled
6 to 8 small parsnips, peeled
8 medium potatoes
1 head cabbage
Sea salt and freshly ground black pepper
White wine vinegar (optional)

Rinse corned beef and place in large saucepan. Cover with water, and simmer over medium-low heat 3 hours. Add prepared vegetables to saucepan and cook until tender. Remove brisket and thinly slice across grain. Place on serving dish with vegetables. Season with salt and pepper to taste. Season individually with vinegar to taste, if desired. Makes 8 servings.

Shepherd's Pie

5 medium russet potatoes, peeled and cubed
4 tablespoons extra-virgin olive oil, divided
1 cup rice milk
1 large onion, chopped, reserve 1 tablespoon, finely chopped
Sea salt and freshly ground pepper to taste

Bottom mixture:
1 teaspoon sea salt
1 clove garlic, minced
5 carrots, sliced into 1/4-inch pieces
1/2 cup celery, diced
1 pound additive-free ground beef
2 tablespoons Worcestershire sauce substitute (optional, see recipe)
1 (8-ounce) can tomato sauce (or see recipe)

To skin tomato, hold on slotted spoon in pot of rapidly boiling water until skin starts to crack and pull away from tomato, about 1 minute or so. Remove, let cool, and discard skin. Bring large saucepan of salted water to boil over medium-high heat. Add potatoes, and continue to cook until tender, about 20 minutes. Drain and mash with 2 tablespoons olive oil and 1 cup of milk, pouring milk in a little at a time until it reaches a thick consistency. Do not add any more milk. Mix in finely 1 tablespoon finely chopped onion. Season with salt and pepper to taste, and set aside. Preheat oven to 375° F. Heat remaining oil in large skillet. Add garlic, chopped onion, carrots, celery and 1 teaspoon salt cook about 6 minutes, stirring frequently. Add ground beef (or meat of choice) into skillet and stir well to combine, breaking up the meat as you stir. Cook an additional 6 to 8 minutes, or until meat is no longer pink. Drain excess fat, then add Worcestershire sauce substitute (if using), and tomato sauce. Bring to boil, reduce heat and simmer uncovered, stirring frequently, until liquid has been absorbed and thickened, about 6 minutes. Spread meat mixture in even layer on bottom of 2-quart casserole dish. Spread layer of mashed potatoes on top, creating "peaks" for better browning. Bake 20 minutes, or until golden brown. Let rest 5 minutes before serving. Serve hot. Makes 6 servings.

Stuffed Cabbage Rolls

2 onions, 1 sliced, 1 chopped
5 tablespoons extra-virgin olive oil
5 cloves garlic, minced
2 green chilies, seeded and chopped
1 (3-inch) piece of fresh ginger, grated
1 pound additive-free ground beef
1/4 teaspoon turmeric
2 teaspoons Garam Masala (see recipe)
1 head savoy cabbage, cored
2 (8-ounce) cans tomato sauce (or see recipe)
2 tablespoons lemon juice
Sea salt and freshly ground pepper to taste
2/3 cup water
Lemon slices, to garnish (optional)

Heat 2 tablespoons oil in large saucepan over medium heat. Add chopped onion and cook 8 minutes, stirring until tender and brown. Add garlic, chilies, and 1/3 of the ginger. Cook 1 minute, then remove with slotted spoon and set aside. Add beef and cook, stirring, until meat is broken up and well browned. Stir in turmeric and Garam Masala. Cook 1 minute, then add onion mixture. Cover and cook 20 to 30 minutes, stirring occasionally, until liquid is absorbed. Set aside and cool. Cook whole cabbage in salted boiling water 8 minutes. Drain and rinse in cold water. Let sit until cool enough to handle, then carefully peel off 12 to 16 outside leaves, being careful to keep them whole. Finely shred rest of cabbage. For sauce, heat remaining oil in a heavy saucepan over medium heat, add sliced onion and cook 5 minutes, stirring frequently, until tender but not brown. Add shredded cabbage, tomato sauce, remaining ginger, lemon juice, salt, pepper and water. Bring to boil, reduce heat to medium-low and simmer 5 minutes. Preheat oven to 375°F. Put 2 tablespoons beef mixture on each cabbage leaf, fold sides in and roll up neatly. Pour a little sauce into bottom of casserole dish. Add cabbage rolls and pour rest of sauce over cabbage rolls. Cover and bake 40 to 50 minutes, until cabbage is tender. Serve hot, garnished with lemon slices. Makes 4 to 6 servings.

Tropical Spiced Steak

1-1/2 pounds additive-free tri-tip or beef steak
2 tablespoons sea salt
1/2 tablespoon freshly ground black pepper
1 tablespoon pure cane dark brown sugar (see note)
1 teaspoon fresh ginger, grated

Tropical barbeque sauce:
1/2 cup additive-free ketchup (see recipe)
1 tablespoon orange juice
2 teaspoons fresh ginger, grated
1 clove garlic, minced
3 teaspoons Coconut Aminos (see note)
1 teaspoon balsamic vinegar
Sea salt and freshly ground pepper to taste

Whisk marinade ingredients together in small bowl, and refrigerate until used. Pat meat dry with paper towel. Mix salt, pepper, brown sugar and ginger together in small bowl. Rub onto both sides of steak, pressing spices gently into flesh. Refrigerate 2 to 3 hours. Remove meat and brush top side with prepared sauce. Place meat top side down on slightly greased hot grill. Brush barbeque sauce on reverse side. Cook 8 minutes per side for medium to medium-rare. Remove and let rest 5 minutes before slicing. For best results, cut in thin slices against the grain. Makes 4 servings.

Dark brown sugar can be replaced with 1/2 cup white sugar and 2 tablespoons corn-free molasses or Yacon syrup for each 1/2 cup.

Coconut Aminos can be substituted for soy sauce in dressings, marinades and other recipes. This product is not derived from the nut of the coconut tree.

Veal Marsala

1 pound additive-free veal cutlets
3/4 teaspoon sea salt
1/4 teaspoon freshly ground black pepper
3/4 cup potato flour
1/4 cup extra-virgin olive oil
2 cloves garlic, minced
1 package (16-ounce) mushrooms, sliced
1 cup dry Marsala wine
1 tablespoon potato starch
1/2 cup beef stock (see recipe)

Sprinkle veal cutlets with salt and pepper. Dredge each cutlet in potato flour and shake off extra. Heat oil in a large skillet over medium-high heat. Add cutlets and cook until brown, about 2 minutes per side. Transfer cutlets to plate and cover. Add garlic to skillet and sauté 1 minute. If necessary, add more oil. Add mushrooms and sauté until tender, about 3 to 5 minutes. Add Marsala wine, reduce heat to medium-low and simmer until liquid reduces by about half. Meanwhile, whisk potato starch into beef stock until dissolved. Add to skillet and whisk constantly until sauce thickens, whisking constantly. Return cutlets to skillet and continue cooking until cutlets are heated through, 1 to 2 minutes. To serve, place cutlet on plate and spoon sauce over top. Makes 4 servings.

Yankee Pot Roast and Vegetables

1 additive-free beef chuck pot roast (2-1/2 pounds)
3 medium baking potatoes, peeled and quartered
2 large carrots, chopped
2 ribs celery, chopped
1 medium onion, quartered
1 large parsnip, chopped
2 bay leaves
1 teaspoon dried rosemary
1/2 teaspoon dried thyme
1/2 cup beef stock (see recipe)
2 tablespoons Coconut Aminos (optional, see note)
Sea salt and freshly ground pepper
2 teaspoons to 2 tablespoons potato starch

Trim excess fat from meat and discard. Cut into serving sized pieces. Sprinkle with salt and pepper. Combine vegetables, bay leaves, rosemary and thyme in slow cooker. Place beef over vegetables. Pour stock and Coconut Aminos (if using) over beef. Cover and cook on low setting 8-1/2 to 9 hours or until beef is fork tender. Remove beef to serving platter. Arrange vegetables around beef. Makes 6 servings.

To thicken gravy, measure juices, and let stand 5 minutes. Skim off and discard fat. Bring to boil in small saucepan. Reduce heat to low and simmer. For each 1 cup of liquid used, you will need 1 tablespoon potato starch. For thinner gravy, use 2 teaspoons potato starch per 1 cup of liquid. Whisk the starch in a small bowl with enough cold water to make it on the runnier side of thick. Mix into gravy, whisking constantly. Turn off heat immediately, and remove from heat source. Continue to whisk until gravy thickens, 1 to 2 more minutes.

Coconut Aminos can be substituted for soy sauce in dressings, marinades and other recipes. This product is not derived from the nut of the coconut tree.

Beverages

Banana Apricot Smoothie ~ 34
Blueberry Smoothie ~ 34
Herbed Tomato Smoothie ~ 35
Hot Chocolate ~ 36
Lime and Mint Drink ~ 37
Sunbutter Banana Smoothie ~ 37

Banana Apricot Smoothie

1-1/2 cups chilled corn-free apricot nectar
3 fresh apricots, seeded and diced (skins on)
2 ounces dried apricots, diced (optional)
2 cups banana slices, frozen
4 dried apricots for garnish (optional)

Combine apricot nectar and fresh apricots in blender. Blend on high speed 15 seconds. Add banana slices and dried apricots, if using, and blend until mixture is smooth. Garnish with dried apricots if desired, and serve immediately. Makes 4 servings.

Blueberry Smoothie

1/2 pear, core removed (skin on)
6 strawberries, tops removed
10 grapes
1 cup blueberries
1/2 kiwi, top and tough, upper center core removed (skin on)
1/2 peach (skin on)
1/2 avocado (seed and skin removed)
1/2 teaspoon green Matcha tea (optional)
1 tablespoon Chia seeds (optional)
1-1/2 cups rice milk

Place all ingredients in blender, starting with fruit, then Matcha tea and Chia, then finally the rice milk. Blend on high speed until mixture is smooth. Liquid at top should be swirling and being drawn back down to bottom. It can take about a minute or so for this to happen depending on the power of your blender and how full the jar is. Garnish with fruit slices if desired, and serve immediately. Keeps several days in the refrigerator. Shake well before use. Makes 4 to 5 servings.

Herbed Tomato Smoothie

1 cup chilled additive-free tomato juice
2/3 cup shelled sunflower seeds
1 tablespoon lemon juice
1/2 cup fresh basil, loosely packed
1/4 cup fresh oregano, loosely packed
1/4 cup fresh parsley, loosely packed
1 large fresh tomato, cored, diced and frozen
Sea salt and freshly ground black pepper to taste

Combine tomato juice, sunflower seeds, lemon juice, basil, oregano and parsley in blender. Blend on high speed 15 seconds. Add frozen tomatoes and blend until mixture is smooth. If it gets too slushy, let sit for several minutes, and blend again. Season to taste with salt and pepper to taste, and serve immediately. Makes 4 servings.

Hot Chocolate

1-1/2 cups rice milk
2 tablespoons Enjoy Life Mini-Chocolate Chips
2 teaspoons Agave nectar
1/4 teaspoon corn-free vanilla

Combine rice milk, chocolate chips, Agave nectar and vanilla in small saucepan over medium-high heat. Stir constantly until chocolate chips have melted, about 3 to 5 minutes. Cool to desired temperature. Makes 2 (6-ounce) servings.

Can be made in larger batches and chilled for chocolate milk. Just be sure to shake well before using!

Beware of adding marshmallows to hot chocolate. They are very risky for hidden allergens.

Hot Chocolate, Thick and Dreamy Version

1-1/2 cups rice milk
6 soft pitted Medjool dates
1-1/2 tablespoons Enjoy Life Mini-Chocolate Chips

Place pitted dates and rice milk in blender or food processor. Blend or process until dates are about as liquefied as you can get them. Don't worry if there are small chunks left. Strain into small saucepan, and add chocolate chips. Stir constantly until chocolate chips have melted, about 3 to 5 minutes. Cool to desired temperature. Makes 2 (6-ounce) servings.

Can be made in larger batches and chilled for chocolate milk. Just be sure to shake well before using!

Beware of adding marshmallows to hot chocolate. They are very risky for hidden allergens.

Lime and Mint Drink

6 tablespoons lime juice
1/4 cup corn-free superfine sugar (see note)
Pinch of sea salt
1 cup fresh mint leaves, packed
Ice cubes
4 to 5 cups cold water
Lime slices and mint leaves to garnish (optional)

Pour lime juice into blender. Add sugar, salt and mint leaves and process until smooth. Strain into pitcher. Cover and refrigerate until cold. This will make the lime juice concentrate. To serve, half-fill 4 to 5 tall glasses with ice cubes. Add a little lime juice concentrate to taste, and top with iced water. Garnish with lime slices and mint leaves if desired, and serve at once. Makes 4 to 5 servings.

Superfine sugar dissolves instantly in liquids. Can be replaced with agave nectar as a sweetener in many recipes.

Sunbutter Banana Smoothie

1 banana (pre-frozen, if desired)
2 tablespoons sunflower seed butter
1 cup rice milk
2 tablespoons corn-free honey (see note)

In a blender, combine banana, sunflower seed butter and rice milk. I like to slice and freeze my bananas ahead of time to make a slushier smoothie. Blend on high speed until mixture is smooth. Pour into glass and drizzle with honey for garnish. Makes 1 serving.

Always use caution when buying honey. Unless you buy certified 100% pure organic, it may contain unlabeled high fructose corn syrup. Honey can be replaced with agave nectar in many recipes.

Breads and Pizza

All-Purpose Flour Blend

2 cups white rice flour
1 cup tapioca starch/flour
1 cup potato starch

Combine thoroughly in large bowl. Store in airtight container until ready for use. Makes 4 cups.

When using the above flour mix in baking, if the amount of guar gum needed isn't listed in the recipe, add the following amounts for 1 cup of flour used:

Cookies ~ 1/4 to 1/2 teaspoon per cup of flour
Cakes and Pancakes ~ 3/4 teaspoon per cup of flour
Muffins and Quick Breads ~ 1 teaspoon per cup of flour
Breads ~ 1-1/2 to 2 teaspoons per cup of flour
Pizza Dough ~ 1 tablespoon per cup of flour

If you purchase a commercial flour blend, read the ingredient list carefully. Some blends contain xanthan gum (which is often derived from corn) or guar gum. Both are used as a thickener and binder. If the blend contains xanthan gum, don't buy if corn allergies are an issue for you. If the blend contains guar gum already, there is no need to add more.

Guar Gum in General

When using guar gum for hot foods such as gravies, stews and sauces, use 1 to 3 teaspoons of guar gum per quart of liquid.

When using guar gum for cold foods, such as salad dressing, ice cream and pudding, use about 1 to 2 teaspoons per quart of liquid.

Banana Bread

1 tablespoon flax seed meal
3 tablespoons warm water
1-1/2 cups all-purpose flour blend (see recipe)
2 teaspoons guar gum (omit if in flour mix)
3/4 teaspoon cream of tartar
1/2 teaspoon baking soda
1/4 teaspoon ground cinnamon
1 cup ripe mashed bananas
3/4 cup pure cane sugar
1/4 cup canola oil (plus more to grease pan)
2 tablespoons rice milk or water

Preheat oven to 350° F. Grease loaf pan(s) with thin layer of oil. Combine flax seed meal and warm water and set aside 10 minutes. In a large bowl, combine flour blend, guar gum (if needed), cream of tartar, baking soda and cinnamon. In another bowl, combine bananas, sugar, oil and flaxseed mixture. Add banana mixture to flour mixture and mix just until moistened. Spoon batter into prepared loaf pan(s).

For one 8 by 4 by 2 inch loaf pan, bake for 50 to 60 minutes
For three 6 by 3 by 2 inch loaf pans, bake for 20 to 25 minutes
For muffins, bake 18 to 20 minutes

Bread should be golden brown on top. It is done when a toothpick inserted in the middle comes out clean.

Braided Sweet Bread

1/2 cup warm water
2 teaspoons plus 1/2 cup pure cane sugar
2-1/4 teaspoons Red Star Active Dry Yeast (the 1/4 ounce size is
        the only one that is corn-free)
2 cups brown rice flour
1/2 cup potato starch
1/2 cup tapioca starch/flour
1 tablespoon guar gum
1 teaspoon sea salt
3 tablespoons canola oil plus more to grease baking sheet
1/2 cup warm rice milk

Egg replacement mixture:
1/4 cup water
1/4 cup canola oil
1-1/2 teaspoons cream of tartar
3/4 teaspoon baking soda

Preheat oven to 350° F. Lightly grease metal baking sheet. In a
small bowl, combine 1/2 cup warm water, 2 teaspoons sugar and
yeast. Cover with damp paper towel and set aside in warm place for
10 minutes. Mixture should foam up about 1-inch high. In large
bowl, mix rice flour, potato starch, tapioca starch/flour, 1/2 cup
sugar, guar gum and salt until well combined. In separate bowl,
whisk egg replacement mixture together. Add to dry ingredients,
add 3 tablespoons canola oil and warm rice milk, and combine. Add
yeast mixture to dough and mix again until dough forms. This could
take up to 10 minutes by hand, really working the dough together
good. It should be soft and sticky. Divide dough into three equal
parts and roll them out into 14-inch ropes. Lay ropes side by side
on baking sheet. Braid the dough starting with the middle rope.
Pinch ends together, turn under and pinch to seal. Cover and let
rise 40 minutes. Place in preheated oven and bake 40 to 45 minutes.
Bread is done when bottom sounds hollow when tapped. Makes 1
loaf.

If yeast mixture does not foam, either it was no good, or the water
was too hot or too cold. Throw out yeast mixture and try again.

Cilantro Black Bean Pizza Topping

1 recipe pizza dough, divided into 2 pizza crusts
1 recipe cilantro-lime pesto
1 tablespoon extra-virgin olive oil
1/2 red onion, thinly sliced
1 red pepper, seeded and thinly sliced
1 can black beans, drained and rinsed
2 cups cubed, cooked chicken breasts

Preheat oven to 450°F. Partially cook pizza dough in preheated oven for 10 minutes. Remove, lightly brush pizza base with 1 tablespoon olive oil. Spread cilantro-lime pesto evenly around pizzas, leaving a 1/2-inch border at edges. Scatter onion, red pepper, beans, and chicken on top. Return to oven, and continue baking 10 to 14 minutes, until bottom of crust browns and topping sizzles. Remove and let stand 2 minutes. Slice and serve hot. Makes 2 pizzas.

Fermented Rice Batter and Lentil Bread

1/3 cup brown lentils
1 cup long grain rice
12 tablespoons water
2 green onions, finely chopped
2 tablespoons cilantro, chopped
1 (1-inch) piece fresh ginger, grated
1 green chili, seeded and chopped
1/2 teaspoon sea salt
About 3 tablespoons water
Extra-virgin olive oil
Cilantro leaves to garnish (optional)

Wash brown lentils and rice thoroughly. Put into separate bowls. Add 2 cups water to each, Soak 3 hours then drain well. Put brown lentils into blender or food processor, add 6 tablespoons water and process until smooth. Puree rice with 6 tablespoons water in the same way. Mix purees together in a large bowl. Cover with a damp cloth and set aside at room temperature about 12 hours. Stir in onion, cilantro, ginger, chili, salt and enough water to make a thin batter. Heat a 6-inch skillet over high heat, brush with a little oil, then pour in 2 to 3 tablespoons batter and spread into a 4-inch circle. Cook about 3 minutes, until browned, turning over after about 1-1/2 minutes. Stack on plate and cover with a dry cloth while cooking remaining bread. Serve warm, garnished with cilantro leaves if desired. Makes 10 to 12 servings.

Hamburger Buns

6 cups all-purpose flour blend (see recipe)
3 tablespoons guar gum (omit if in flour mix)
1 tablespoon Red Star Active Dry Yeast (the 1/4 ounce size is the
    only one that is corn-free)
2-1/2 cups warm water
2 tablespoons pure cane sugar
1 tablespoon sea salt
5 tablespoons canola oil plus more to grease baking sheet

In small bowl, whisk yeast together with warm water. Cover and let
stand in warm area until foamy, about 10 minutes. In large bowl,
blend guar gum (if needed) into all-purpose flour blend. Do not add
if already in flour blend. Combine yeast mixture, sugar, salt and oil
in with the flour, mixing well until a sticky dough forms. Cover and
let stand for 10 minutes. Mix for several more minutes, folding over
and beating down dough as you mix. Cover and let stand until
dough double in size.

Form into balls and place on lightly oiled baking sheet. Squash balls
down with the palm of your hand. If they spring back up, wait a few
minutes and squash them again. Cover with greased plastic wrap
and let rise 1 hour. Preheat oven to 350°F. Bake 18 to 20 minutes.
Makes roughly 12 to 15 buns, depending on size.

See All-Purpose Flour Blend in "Breads and Pizza" section. You
can also shape these into hot-dog buns and adjust the cooking time
to account for the smaller thickness.

High-Protein Flour Blend

1-1/4 cups bean flour or chickpea flour
1 cup potato starch
1 cup tapioca starch/flour
1 cup white rice flour

Combine thoroughly in large bowl. Store in airtight container until
ready for use. Makes 4-1/4 cups.

Pizza Dough

2-1/2 cups high-protein flour blend (see recipe)
1/2 cup millet flour
1 tablespoon guar gum (omit if in flour mix)
1 teaspoon sea salt
5 teaspoons Red Star Active Dry Yeast (the 1/4 ounce size is the
        only one that is corn-free)
1-1/3 cups warm water
2 tablespoons extra-virgin olive oil
1 tablespoon corn-free honey (see note)
1 teaspoon apple cider vinegar

Preheat oven to 450° F. If using pizza stone, place it on lowest rack
before preheating oven. In large bowl with heavy-duty mixer,
combine high-protein flour blend, millet flour, guar gum (if needed)
and salt. Blend well. Add yeast and blend. In small bowl, combine
water, oil, honey and vinegar. Add to dry ingredients. Beat 3 to 5
minutes, or until the dough thickens. You don't need to let this
dough rise; it rises nicely in oven. Scoop half of dough onto lightly
oiled pizza pan. Cover with lightly oiled plastic wrap. Use hands to
gently press dough into a 12-inch circle, creating rim of dough
around edge of pizza. Repeat with remaining pizza dough and pizza
pan. Top with favorite pizza toppings. Bake 20 to 24 minutes,
depending on thickness, until bottom of crust browns. Remove and
let stand 2 minutes. Slice and serve hot. Makes two (12-inch) pizzas.

Always use caution when buying honey. Unless you buy certified
100% pure organic, it may contain unlabeled high fructose corn
syrup. Honey can be replaced with agave nectar in many recipes.

Roasted Tomato and Zucchini Pizza Topping

1 recipe pizza dough
6 cups cherry tomatoes, stemmed and halved
2 small zucchini (about 1 pound), cut into 1/2-inch pieces
2 shallots halved and sliced thin
3 cloves garlic, sliced thin
3 tablespoons extra-virgin olive oil
1 tablespoon balsamic vinegar
1 teaspoon pure cane sugar
1/8 teaspoon red pepper flakes (optional)
1/2 teaspoon sea salt
1/4 teaspoon freshly ground pepper
3 tablespoons fresh basil, chopped

Place oven racks to lower middle and upper middle positions.
Preheat oven to 350° F. Put tomatoes, zucchini, shallots, garlic, 2
tablespoons oil, vinegar, sugar, red pepper flakes (if used), salt and
pepper in a bowl and toss well. Spread vegetables out over 2
rimmed baking sheets. Roast without stirring until tomato skins
have shriveled slightly, and shallot edges begin to brown, 35 to 40
minutes, rotating baking sheets halfway through baking. Let cool
slightly. Increase oven to 450°F. Partially cook pizza dough in
preheated oven for 10 minutes. Remove, lightly brush pizza base
with 1 tablespoon olive oil. Scatter topping evenly over pizzas,
leaving a 1/2-inch border at edges. Return to oven, and bake 10 to
14 minutes, until bottom of crust browns and topping sizzles.
Remove, let stand 2 minutes. Slice and serve hot. Makes 2 pizzas.

Topping Variations

Roasted tomato and mushrooms: Omit vinegar. Substitute 1 pound
white or fancy mushrooms for zucchini.

Roasted tomatoes and eggplant: Omit vinegar. Substitute 1
eggplant, diced into 1/2-inch pieces, for the zucchini and 1
tablespoon fresh chopped mint for the basil.

Self-Rising Flour Blend

1-1/4 cups white sorghum flour
1-1/4 cups white rice flour
1/2 cup tapioca starch/flour
2 teaspoons guar gum
2 teaspoons cream of tartar
1 teaspoon baking soda
1/2 teaspoon sea salt

Mix thoroughly, and store in airtight container. Use this blend for muffins, scones, cakes, cupcakes or any recipe that uses baking powder for leavening.

Vegetable Pizza Topping

1 tablespoon extra-virgin olive oil
2 cloves garlic, minced
1 cup carrot, grated
1/8 cup fresh basil, chopped finely
2 medium vine-ripened tomatoes, cut into 1/4-inch slices
1 small zucchini, thinly sliced
1 cup asparagus pieces, about 1-1/2-inch long
8 black brined olives, halved and pitted (see note)

Preheat oven to 375° F. Heat oil in a small skillet over medium heat. Add leek and garlic and sauté, stirring occasionally, until soft, about 5 minutes. Stir in carrot and cook 1 minute longer. Set aside to cool. Spoon leek and carrot mixture onto middle of pizza base and spread to within 3/4-inch of the edge. Sprinkle with fresh basil. Arrange the sliced zucchini over the center of the pizza in a single layer. Arrange tomato slices around outside edge. Place asparagus pieces on top of tomatoes. Scatter olives over top. Bake according to original pizza crust recipe, or until crust is cooked and topping starts to brown, about 25 minutes. Slice and serve immediately. Makes enough topping for 2 pizzas.

Make sure the olives are brined with white wine vinegar, not distilled white vinegar, which may contain corn or gluten.

White Bean Pizza Topping

1 recipe pizza dough
1 recipe caramelized onions
1 (15-ounce) can white navy beans
1 tablespoon extra-virgin olive oil
1 clove garlic, minced
1 teaspoon dried rosemary

Preheat oven to 450°F. In food processor or blender, puree together 1/2 cup of beans, oil, garlic, and rosemary. Remove and mix in remaining beans. Partially cook pizza dough in preheated oven for 10 minutes. Remove, lightly brush pizza base with 1 tablespoon olive oil. Spread white bean mixture evenly around pizzas, leaving a 1/2-inch border at edges. Top with caramelized onions. Return to oven, and continue baking 10 to 14 minutes, until bottom of crust browns and topping sizzles. Remove and let stand 2 minutes. Slice and serve hot. Makes 2 pizzas.

Breakfast

Banana Donuts ~ 50
Buckwheat Pancakes ~ 50
Granola Bars ~ 51
Muesli ~ 52
Oatmeal ~ 53
Oatmeal Raisin Breakfast Treats ~ 54
Pull-Apart Honey Rolls ~ 55
Quinoa Cereal with Fresh Fruit ~ 56
Rice and Blueberries ~ 56
Rice Flour Pancakes ~ 57
Waffles ~ 58

Banana Donuts

2 large bananas (peeled and mashed)
1-1/2 cups golden flax seeds
1 tablespoon pure cane sugar (optional)
1/2 teaspoon cinnamon (optional)
Agave nectar (optional)
1/3 cup Chocolate Maple Cookie Glaze (optional, see recipe)

In food processor, grind flax seeds to a fine powder. Pour ground flax seeds into bowl with mashed bananas and mix until evenly coated. Depending on how firm you like your donuts, adjust the amount of flax seeds. As flax seeds get absorbed into the bananas, the mixture will get harder and firm up. Roll into a long tube shape, then slice and form into donuts. If using coating, mix sugar and cinnamon in a small bowl. Lightly drizzle donuts with agave nectar, then sprinkle with sugar cinnamon mixture. Or if desired, skip the agave nectar and sugar cinnamon mixture, and coat with chocolate maple cookie glaze instead. Makes 2 large donuts, or 4 mini-donuts.

Buckwheat Pancakes

2 teaspoons lemon juice
3 tablespoons extra-virgin olive oil
2 tablespoons maple syrup
2 cups buckwheat flour
1/2 teaspoon cream of tartar
1/2 teaspoon baking soda
1/2 teaspoon sea salt
Maple syrup or blueberry sauce (optional, see recipe)

Preheat skillet over medium heat. Mix rice milk, lemon juice, oil and maple syrup in large bowl. In separate bowl, mix together buckwheat, cream of tartar, baking soda and salt. Whisk ingredients together until just mixed. Allow mixture to stand 2 to 3 minutes until it rises. Scoop batter onto skillet, forming 3 to 4-inch pancakes. Cook until bubbles form on surface and batter sets around edges, then flip and cook for another couple of minutes. Serve immediately with topping, if desired. Makes 8 to 12 pancakes.

Granola Bars

4 cups gluten-free rolled oats
1/2 cup safflower oil
1/4 cup pure cane sugar
1/2 cup brown rice syrup
3/4 teaspoon dried ginger
1/2 teaspoon sea salt
3/4 cup dried fruit (optional)

Preheat oven to 300°F. In an oven-safe bowl, mix together oats, oil, sugar, ginger and salt. The mixture will be moist and crumbly. Cook on middle rack 15 minutes. Stir, and cook again another 15 minutes. Stir again and cook 5 minutes. The sugars will have caramelized and turned a light brown color. Line a cookie sheet with parchment paper. Remove bowl from oven and stir again. If using dried fruit, toss into mixture, working quickly before it cools. Use spatula to gently shape mixture into a rectangle in the middle of the parchment paper, patting the mixture down firmly as you do so. Allow to cool, then cut into bars. Will keep several weeks in airtight container in refrigerator. Makes 16 to 24 bars, depending on size.

Cinnamon Raisin Granola Bars

Follow recipe above, but before baking, add 1 teaspoon cinnamon to oat mixture. After the final baking, sprinkle top of mixture with 1/2 cup raisins. Toss into mixture, working quickly before it cools. Shape into rectangle, allow to cool, and cut into bars. Will keep several weeks in airtight container in refrigerator. Makes 16 to 24 bars, depending on size.

Muesli

3 cups gluten-free rolled oats
3 cups corn-free, gluten-free crispy rice cereal
1/2 cup diced dried apples or pears
1/2 cup golden raisins
1/2 cup pure cane dark brown sugar (see note)
1/4 cup sunflower seeds, shelled
1/4 cup pumpkin seeds, shelled

Fruit suggestions:
2 pineapple rings, chopped
1 medium banana, sliced
1 small nectarine or peach, sliced
1/2 medium apple or pear, grated
1/2 medium mango, diced
1/2 cup stewed plums, prunes or rhubarb
1/2 seasonal berries or pitted cherries

Liquid suggestions:
1/3 cup apple juice
1/3 cup grape juice
1/3 cup orange juice
1/3 cup pear juice
1/3 cup apricot nectar
1/3 cup prune juice
1/3 cup rice milk

Combine first 8 ingredients in a large bowl. Transfer mixture to a large glass jar with a tight fitting lid. Store in a cool, dry place. Makes 7 cups.

For a balanced breakfast serve Muesli with liquid and fruit of choice. Dark brown sugar can be replaced with 1/2 cup white sugar and 2 tablespoons corn-free molasses or Yacon syrup for each 1/2 cup.

Oatmeal

2 cups water
1 cup gluten-free rolled oats
1/4 teaspoon sea salt

Add-In Suggestions:
Raisins (add to water so they plump up)
Dried cranberries (add to water to plump up)
Any other dried fruit (add to water to plump up)
Pineapple bits
Sliced bananas
Blueberries
Sliced strawberries
Sliced soft peaches
Maple syrup
Diced apple and dash of cinnamon (add apple to water to soften)
Additive-free apple butter (see recipe)
Sunflower seed butter
Frozen berries

In small saucepan, bring salt and water to boil. Add oatmeal and cook until it begins to thicken, 1 to 2 minutes. Reduce heat and simmer 10 minutes, stirring occasionally. Add desired mix-in ingredients, stir, and pour into 4 bowls. Serve hot. Makes 4 servings.

Oatmeal Raisin Breakfast Treats

2/3 cup pure cane sugar
2/3 cup pure cane dark brown sugar (see note)
1/3 cup additive-free applesauce
1/2 cup Spectrum brand palm oil shortening
1-1/2 teaspoons corn-free vanilla
1-1/4 teaspoon baking soda
1/2 teaspoon cream of tartar
1-1/2 teaspoon cinnamon
1 teaspoon sea salt
2-3/4 cups gluten-free rolled oats
2-1/2 cups all-purpose flour blend (see recipe)
2 tablespoons guar gum (omit if in flour mix)
1/4 cup dried dates, pulsed in food processor
2 tablespoons flax seed meal
1/2 cup hot water
1 cup raisins

Preheat oven to 375° F. In small bowl, whisk together 2 tablespoons flax seed meal and water. Let thicken for 10 minutes. In large bowl, combine sugar, dark brown sugar, applesauce, vanilla and shortening. Add thickened flax mixture and blend well. In separate bowl, whisk together baking soda, cream of tartar, cinnamon, salt, oats, guar gum (if needed), dates and flour blend. Slowly add dry mix into wet ingredients, mixing well. Stir in raisins. Spoon dough by 2 tablespoons each onto insulated baking sheet, 2-inches apart. Bake 10 minutes, or until center is done. Remove and cool on wire racks. They freeze well in an airtight container. Makes roughly 3 dozen treats.

Dark brown sugar can be replaced with 1/2 cup white sugar and 2 tablespoons corn-free molasses or Yacon syrup for each 1/2 cup.

Pull-Apart Honey Rolls

4 cups all-purpose flour blend, more for dusting (see recipe)
1 tablespoons plus 1 teaspoon guar gum (omit if in flour mix)
1-1/4 teaspoon cream of tartar
1/2 teaspoon baking soda
1/2 teaspoon sea salt
3 teaspoons corn-free yeast
1/2 cup canola oil
2 tablespoons corn-free honey (see note)
6 tablespoons additive-free applesauce
2 cups warm rice milk

Lightly grease two 8 by 8 inch baking pans. In large bowl, combine flour, guar gum (if needed), cream of tartar, baking soda, salt, and yeast, and mix until combined. Add oil, honey and applesauce and mix until dough starts to stick together. Slowly add rice milk while continuing to mix. Once mixture has started to form, continue to mix for about another 10 minutes. The dough should be thick and smooth, but tacky to touch. If it's too wet, add flour mixture 1 tablespoon full at a time and mix until right consistency. Put dough on floured surface and divide evenly into 24 balls. If necessary, roll ball in flour to prevent from sticking together. Arrange balls on prepared pans, spacing them evenly. Cover pans with plastic wrap, and place in warm spot. Allow dough to rise 30 minutes, or until rolls are double their size and touching one another. While rolls are rising, preheat oven to 375°F. Bake 18 to 20 minutes until lightly browned, rotating once while baking. Makes 24 rolls.

Always use caution when buying honey. Unless you buy certified 100% pure organic, it may contain unlabeled high fructose corn syrup. Honey can be replaced with agave nectar in many recipes.

Quinoa Cereal with Fresh Fruit

1/2 cup quinoa
1 cups water
Sea salt to taste

Topping:
1/2 cup gluten-free rolled oats
1/2 cup blueberries
2 tablespoons shelled pumpkin or sunflower seeds
1/2 cup rice milk mixed with 1 teaspoon corn-free honey (see note)
Add any of your favorite fresh fruits in season

Rinse quinoa and place in small with water and salt, cover and bring
to boil. Reduce heat to low, cover, and simmer 15 minutes. Divide
quinoa between two bowls, adding one-half of the rolled oats on
top of each. Top each bowl with half of the blueberries, and
pumpkin or sunflower seeds. Serve immediately with rice milk and
honey. Makes 2 servings.

See caution on buying honey at bottom of page.

Rice and Blueberries

1 cup cooked long grain white rice
1/2 cup blueberries
1/4 teaspoon nutmeg
3 teaspoons corn-free honey (see note)
1/2 cup hot rice milk

Spoon rice and blueberries into 2 bowls. Sprinkle with honey and
nutmeg. Pour hot rice milk over top and serve. If using leftover
rice, warm rice, rice milk and honey in a saucepan before adding
blueberries. Makes 2 servings.

Always use caution when buying honey. Unless you buy certified
100% pure organic, it may contain unlabeled high fructose corn
syrup. Honey can be replaced with agave nectar in many recipes.

Rice Flour Pancakes

1 cup white rice flour
3/4 tablespoon corn-free honey (see note)
1 teaspoon cream of tartar
1/2 teaspoon baking soda
1/8 teaspoon sea salt
1 cup of rice milk
2 tablespoons extra-virgin olive oil
Maple syrup (optional)
Blueberry sauce (optional, see recipe)

Combine rice flour, cream of tartar, baking soda and salt in bowl. Add honey, rice milk and oil. Mix well, then spread into 3-inch pancakes on a lightly greased skillet over medium-high heat. Cook until pancake sets and bottom begins to brown. Flip and cook other side until lightly browned on bottom. Serve immediately with slightly warmed maple syrup or blueberry sauce, if desired. Makes 3 to 4 servings.

Always use caution when buying honey. Unless you buy certified 100% pure organic, it may contain unlabeled high fructose corn syrup. Honey can be replaced with agave nectar in many recipes.

Waffles

2 cups all-purpose flour blend (see recipe)
2 tablespoons rice protein powder
1 teaspoon cream of tartar
1/2 teaspoon baking soda
2 tablespoons pure cane sugar
3 tablespoons canola oil plus more for small spray bottle
1 tablespoon apple cider vinegar
1-1/2 cups rice milk (plus more, if needed)
1 teaspoon corn-free vanilla
Maple syrup (optional)
Blueberry sauce (optional, see recipe)

Preheat waffle iron and mist surface with canola oil. In medium mixing bowl, combine flour, protein powder, cream of tartar, baking soda and sugar. Add vinegar, oil, rice milk and vanilla and mix well. If mixture is too thick, add more rice milk. Pour enough batter to fill wells and cook according to manufacturer instructions. Serve warm, with lightly heated maple syrup or blueberry sauce. Leftovers freeze well. Makes 4 waffles.

Cakes, Cookies and Muffins

Banana Muffins

1 tablespoon flax seed meal
3 tablespoons warm water
1-1/3 cups all-purpose flour blend (see recipe)
1-1/3 teaspoons guar gum (omit if in flour mix)
3/4 cup gluten-free rolled oats
1/3 cup pure cane sugar
1 teaspoon cream of tartar
1/2 teaspoon baking soda
1/4 teaspoons sea salt
3/4 cups rice milk
3/4 cups mashed banana (about 3 medium)
1/4 cups canola oil plus extra to grease muffin tins
1 teaspoon corn-free vanilla
1/2 cups Enjoy Life mini-chocolate chips (optional)

Preheat oven to 375°F. In small bowl, combine flax seed meal and water, and let set to thicken for 10 minutes. Lightly grease muffin tins with extra canola oil. In mixing bowl, combine flour, guar gum (if needed), oats, sugar, cream of tartar, baking soda and salt. Mix well. Add flaxseed meal mixture, milk, oil, banana and vanilla extract (and cocoa nibs, if using) to dry mixture. With a spoon, mix wet ingredients into dry until moistened. Fill muffin tins 3/4 full. Bake at 375°F for 18 to 20 minutes. For mini-muffins, bake 8 to 10 minutes. Remove from oven and let cool slightly in pan. Remove from pan. Serve warm, or cool completely and transfer to plastic container and freeze. Makes 12 to 24 muffins, depending on size.

Carrot Cake

3/4 cup pure cane sugar
1/4 cup canola oil
3/4 cup additive-free applesauce
3/4 teaspoon corn-free vanilla
1/2 teaspoon cream of tartar
1-1/4 teaspoon baking soda
3/4 cup all-purpose flour blend (see recipe)
3/4 teaspoon guar gum (omit if in flour mix)
1/2 cup tapioca flour
1-1/2 teaspoon cinnamon
1/2 teaspoon sea salt
3/4 raisins
1/2 cup sunflower seeds, shelled
2-1/4 cup carrots, grated
1/4 cup pineapple bits

Preheat the oven to 350°F. Lightly grease 8 by8-inch square pan, or 9-inch round pan. In mixer, beat sugar, oil and applesauce together. Add vanilla. In a large bowl, mix together cream of tartar, baking soda, flour blend, tapioca flour, guar gum (if needed), cinnamon and salt. Add wet ingredients to dry ingredients. Stir in raisins and sunflower seeds. Fold in carrots and pineapple, taking care not to over mix, and pour in cake pan. Bake 35 to 45 minutes, or until a toothpick comes out clean. Allow cake to cool completely in pans set over a wire rack. Makes 10 servings.

Cinnamon Raisin Cake

1 cup pure cane sugar
1/2 cup Spectrum brand palm oil shortening
1-1/2 cups water
1-1/2 teaspoons sea salt
1/2 cup raisins
1 teaspoon cinnamon
1-1/2 teaspoon nutmeg
1 teaspoon ground cloves
2 cups all-purpose flour blend (see recipe)
1-1/2 teaspoons guar gum (omit if in flour mix)
1 teaspoon baking soda
1 tablespoon warm water

Preheat oven to 350°F. In medium saucepan, add sugar, shortening, salt, water, raisins, cinnamon, cloves and nutmeg. Bring to a boil, stirring gently. Remove from heat and let stand until cool. Dissolve baking soda in 1 tablespoon warm water and add to mixture. If guar gum is needed, blend in with flour in separate bowl. Slowly add flour mixture to wet ingredients and stir until well blended. Lightly grease a 7-1/2 by 10-inch pan or for a slightly higher cake, use a 9-inch round pan. Add batter, and bake 30 minutes. This makes a really moist cake that needs no frosting.

Gingerbread Cookies

2 cups brown rice flour
1/4 cup tapioca starch, plus extra for dusting
1/3 cup pure cane sugar
1/3 cup pure cane dark brown sugar (see note)
1/4 teaspoon baking soda
1/4 teaspoon guar gum
1/4 teaspoon dried ginger
1/2 teaspoon cinnamon
1/2 teaspoon sea salt
2 tablespoons grape seed oil
1-1/2 tablespoons corn-free molasses (see note)
1/2 cup rice milk

Preheat oven to 375° F. In a large bowl, combine the first nine ingredients, and blend together well. Whisk the remaining three ingredients together in a separate bowl. Add wet ingredients into the dry ingredients, and mix well, until a clean ball is formed. Dough may appear a little dry at first, but will form nicely after kneading it a couple of
minutes. With a little bit of tapioca starch on your hands, roll the dough into little balls about 1-1/2-inches wide. Flatten them with a lightly dusted rolling pin to about 1/8-inch thickness and place on a well-greased cookie sheet. Bake for 12 to 15 minutes. Let cool about five minutes on the cookie sheet, and then transfer to a cooling rack. Makes 12 to 18 cookies, depending on size.

Dark brown sugar can be replaced with 1/2 cup white sugar and 2 tablespoons corn-free molasses or Yacon syrup for each 1/2 cup.

Can be decorated with frosting once cooled. See Sugar Cookie Frosting recipe in Fillings, Frostings and Glazes section.

Oatmeal Applesauce Cookies

1 tablespoon flax seed meal
3 tablespoons warm water
1/4 cup canola oil
2/3 cup pure cane dark brown sugar (see note)
1/4 teaspoon baking soda
1/2 teaspoon cinnamon
1/2 cup additive-free applesauce
1-1/4 cup all-purpose flour blend (see recipe)
3/4 teaspoon guar gum (omit if in flour blend)
1-1/4 cup gluten-free rolled oats
1/2 cup Enjoy Life mini-chocolate chips
1/3 cup sunflower seeds (optional)

Preheat oven to 375°F. Combine flaxseed meal and warm water in small bowl and set aside. In large bowl, beat oil and brown sugar together until combined. Scrape down sides of bowl. Add baking soda and cinnamon and mix well. Scrape down sides of the bowl again. Add applesauce and flaxseed meal mixture and beat until well combined. If guar gum is needed, mix in with flour in separate bowl. Add to wet ingredients and beat until flour is incorporated into dough. Mix in oats and cocoa nibs. Using a teaspoon, drop dough onto ungreased cookie sheet. Bake 8 to 10 minutes. Transfer to cooling rack and let cool. Makes about 2 dozen cookies.

Dark brown sugar can be replaced with 1/2 cup white sugar and 2 tablespoons corn-free molasses or Yacon syrup for each 1/2 cup.

Shortbread Cookies

1-1/2 cups Spectrum brand palm oil shortening, chilled
1 cup plus 3 tablespoons pure cane sugar, divided
2 tablespoons flax seed meal plus 3/8 cup <u>hot</u> water
2 teaspoons anise seeds
4 cups all-purpose flour blend, extra to dust cookie cutters (see
        recipe)
1-1/2 teaspoons guar gum (omit if in flour mix)
1 teaspoon cream of tartar
1/2 teaspoon baking soda
1/2 teaspoon sea salt
3 tablespoons brandy or corn-free apple juice
1-1/2 teaspoon cinnamon

Preheat oven to 350 ° F. In small bowl, mix flax seed meal and 3/8
cup hot water together and let sit for 5 minutes to set and become
gel-like. With an electric beater, cream together chilled palm
shortening and 1 cup sugar. Add gelled flax seed mixture, anise
seeds, and blend well. In a separate bowl, sift together flour, guar
gum if needed, cream of tartar, baking soda and salt. Add to
creamed mixture along with apple juice. Mix thoroughly until dough
stiffens. Roll out cookie dough to 1/2-inch thickness, and using
flour dusted cookie cutters, cut into desired shapes. Combine
remaining 3 tablespoons sugar with cinnamon, and sprinkle tops of
cookies with mixture. Place cookies on ungreased cookie sheet and
bake for approximately 10 minutes, or until the tops of the cookies
are just firm to the touch. Allow to cool on wire rack. Makes 4 to 6
dozen cookies, depending upon size of cookie cutters you use.

Candy and Desserts

Baked Apples ~ 67
Banana Mango Pudding ~ 67
Bread Pudding ~ 68
Candied Jalapenos ~ 69
Cherry Fig Bars ~ 70
Chocolate Covered Bananas ~ 71
Chocolate Covered Raisins ~ 71
Figs with Orange Ginger Sauce ~ 72
Lime Parfait ~ 73
Sesame Sun-Bars ~ 74
Strawberry Tea Cakes ~ 75

Baked Apples

4 large, tart apples
2 tablespoons raisins
1/2 cup pure cane dark brown sugar (see note)
1 teaspoon cinnamon
1 cup water
3 tablespoons cream sherry

Preheat oven to 375°F. Core the apples, leaving 1/2-inch at the bottom. Mix raisins, sugar and cinnamon together and fill apples with mixture. Place in shallow glass baking dish, and add water and sherry. Bake 30 to 40 minutes, until soft but not mushy, basting several times with the cooking juices. Serve in bowls, and spoon some of the reserved baking liquid over the tops. Makes 4 servings.

Dark brown sugar can be replaced with 1/2 cup white sugar and 2 tablespoons corn-free molasses or Yacon syrup for each 1/2 cup.

Banana Mango Pudding

1 large mango, ripe
2-1/2 medium bananas, ripe to over-ripe
1/2 sliced banana for top
Cinnamon (optional)
Fresh berries (optional)

Combine the first two ingredients in a blender until nice and creamy. Serve in bowls with sliced banana on top. Add cinnamon or fresh berries on top instead of bananas if desired. Makes 4 servings.

Bread Pudding

6 cups of bread cut into 1-inch cubes (see recipe)
3 cups rice milk
1/2 cup pure cane light brown sugar
1/4 cup arrowroot starch / flour
2 teaspoons corn-free vanilla
1 teaspoon ground cinnamon
1/4 cup Spectrum brand palm oil shortening
1/2 cup raisins

Preheat oven to 400° F. In a small bowl, combine cinnamon and arrowroot. Place in a saucepan with rice milk, and whisk together over medium-high heat. Add sugar and vanilla and whisk until combined. Add shortening, and continue to whisk until shortening is melted and the sauce is slightly thickened. Place bread cubes and raisins in a large bowl, and pour hot pudding mixture over the top. Toss gently to coat all the bread cubes. Let bread absorb pudding mixture for 2 minutes. Stir again. Carefully mixture into oven-safe glass baking dish and place in center of the oven. Bake 20 to 25 minutes. Remove from oven, and let stand 15 minutes before serving. Serve warm. Refrigerate any leftovers. Makes 10 to 12 servings.

Candied Jalapenos

3 pounds fresh jalapeno peppers, washed
2 cups apple cider vinegar
6 cups pure cane sugar
1/2 teaspoons turmeric
1/2 teaspoons celery seed
3 teaspoons garlic powder
1 teaspoon cayenne pepper

Remove stems from jalapenos and discard stems. Slice peppers into uniform 1/8-inch rounds. Set aside. In large saucepan over high heat, bring vinegar, sugar, turmeric, celery seed, garlic and cayenne pepper to boil. Reduce heat to medium-low and simmer 5 minutes. Add pepper slices and simmer 4 minutes. Using slotted spoon, transfer peppers into clean, sterile canning jars within 1/4-inch of upper rim. Turn heat up under saucepan with syrup and bring to full boil. Boil for 6 minutes. Use ladle to pour boiling syrup into jars over jalapeno slices. Insert butter knife to bottom of jar two or three times to release trapped pockets of air. Adjust level of the syrup if necessary. Wipe rims of jars with clean, damp paper towel and cover with new two-piece lids to finger-tip tightness. If you do not want to go through the canning process, you can simply put the jars in your refrigerator and store them there.

To can, place jars in a canner and cover with water by 2-inches. Bring water to a full rolling boil. When it reaches a full boil, set timer for 10 minutes for half-pints or 15 minutes for pints. When timer goes off, use canning tongs to transfer the jars to cooling rack. Leave to cool, undisturbed, for 24 hours. When fully cooled, wipe with clean, damp washcloth, then label. Allow to set for at least two weeks, but preferably a month before eating. Makes about 9 half-pint jars.

Cherry Fig Bars

1-1/4 cup sunflower seeds, shelled
3/4 cup pumpkin seeds, shelled
1/4 cup ground flax seed meal
Zest from 2 lemons
1-1/4 cups dried figs, stems removed and diced
2 tablespoon to 1/4 cup agave nectar (depends on dryness)
2 tablespoons tahini
1 cup dried tart cherries, unsweetened

In a food processor, combine seeds and flax seed meal, and process until it begins to stick to sides. Be careful not to over process, you want it to remain lumpy, not smooth and creamy. Add lemon zest and figs, and process again until mixture resembles a coarse meal. Add remaining ingredients and process briefly to chop cherries and create a moist dough (it will form a ball). Pinch a bit of mixture between your fingers. If it sticks together and feels slightly moist, it's ready. Turn mixture into pan lined with plastic wrap, and press down firmly. The mixture should be very compact and solid. Refrigerate until firm, about 1 hour. Cut into bars and store in an airtight container in refrigerator, or wrap each bar individually in plastic wrap. The bars will keep refrigerated up to 2 weeks. They freeze well too. Makes about 10 to 12 bars.

Chocolate Covered Bananas

3 ripe bananas, sliced and frozen
1/2 cup corn-free, gluten-free crispy rice cereal
1/4 cup flax seed meal
2 tablespoons pumpkin seeds, crumbled in food processor
3/4 cup Enjoy Life mini-chocolate chips
2 teaspoons Spectrum brand palm oil shortening
Popsicle sticks (can be found at many craft stores)

Peel and slice bananas into roughly 2-inch chunks. Place flat side
down on lightly greased plate, insert popsicle sticks, and freeze for
about 30 minutes. Place cereal, crumbled pumpkin seeds and flax
meal together in a sealable plastic baggie. Flatten with rolling pin
until rice crispy cereal is fine and crumbly, and mixture has blended
together. Empty into small bowl. In small saucepan over medium
heat, whisk melt chocolate chips and shortening together. Reduce
heat to medium-low, and keep whisk handy. Remove bananas from
freezer, dip into chocolate, and allow excess chocolate to drip into
saucepan. Dip in cereal coating, and roll to coat. Repeat until all
bananas are used. If not eaten immediately, return to freezer until
frozen. Once frozen, wrap each with plastic wrap and tie top closed
around popsicle stick, and return to freezer.

Chocolate Covered Raisins

1 bag (10-ounces) Enjoy Life mini-chocolate chips
2 teaspoon Spectrum brand palm oil shortening
1 cup raisins

Line cookie sheet with parchment paper. Combine chocolate chips
and shortening in a microwavable bowl. Heat for 30 seconds, then
remove and stir. Continue until all chocolate is melted and smooth.
Add raisins and mix until coated. Using a slotted spoon, remove the
coated raisins. Placed chocolate covered raisin clusters on
parchment and let cool to harden. Once cooled, break apart pieces
if needed. Yield depends on size of clusters.

Figs with Orange Ginger Sauce

1 cup orange juice
1 tablespoon fresh ginger, grated
1 star anise
12 fresh figs
Fresh mint leaves for garnish (optional)

In medium saucepan, bring orange juice, ginger, and star anise to boil, then reduce heat to medium-low and simmer 20 minutes, or until volume is reduced by half so it will stick to figs. While sauce is simmering, cut figs in half from stem to stem, and set aside in covered dish. Strain sauce, discarding all but liquid. Chill in refrigerator 1 hour. Sauce should thicken a bit more as it chills. Arrange figs on plates and drizzle with sauce. Garnish with fresh mint leaves if desired. Makes 4 servings.

Lime Parfait

2/3 cup Udi's Au Naturel Granola
Lime zest from 1 lime (reserve lime)
5 dates, seeds removed and quartered
1/3 cup sunflower seeds, shelled

Lime cream:
2 medium avocados, seeds and skin removed
Lime zest from 1 lime (reserve lime)
4 to 5 tablespoons lime juice
1/3 cup agave nectar

Fresh fruit for garnish (optional)

Place granola, zest from first lime, dates and sunflower seeds in food processor and process until it resembles wet sand. Transfer to small bowl and set aside. Place avocados, zest from second lime, 4 tablespoons lime juice (5 if you prefer it tart), and agave nectar in food processor and process until creamy.

In either two regular sized, or four small parfait glasses (any type of short clear class with a wide top will work), start your layers with 2 tablespoons lime cream, then a layer of granola date crumble, then more lime cream, and so on until you have several layers and have used up all the lime cream. Sprinkle top with extra granola crumble, and garnish with fresh fruit if desired. Makes 2 to 4 servings, depending on size.

Sesame Sun-Bars

1/2 cup sunflower seeds, shelled
1/4 cup pumpkin seeds, shelled
1 tablespoon flax seed meal
1/2 cup sesame seeds
1-1/2 cups dates, pitted
1-1/2 cups raisins
1/8 teaspoon sea salt

Place all ingredients in a food processor. Pulse just until mixture holds together when pressed. Scoop into a 9-inch square pan, and refrigerate until thoroughly chilled, about 1 hour. Cut into squares to serve. Makes 20 to 30 bars, depending how wide you slice them.

Strawberry Tea Cakes

1 cup strawberries, trimmed and diced into small pieces
3/4 cup millet flour
1 cup potato starch
1/2 cup tapioca starch
1 cup pure cane sugar
1/2 teaspoon cream of tartar
1/4 teaspoon baking soda
1 teaspoon sea salt
1 teaspoon guar gum
3/4 cup Spectrum brand palm oil shortening, plus extra to grease
        sheet
1/4 cup cold rice milk

Preheat oven to 350° F. Prepare strawberries, and set aside. In a large bowl, whisk together millet flour, potato starch, tapioca starch, sugar, cream of tartar, baking soda, salt and guar gum. Cut shortening into dry mix with pastry cutter. Add prepared strawberries, and toss lightly to combine. Slowly stir rice milk into dough, taking care not to over mix, but make sure there are no dry lumps. Scrape dough from sides and blend into mix. Dough should pull away from bowl and form a soft ball. Spoon by heaping tablespoons onto lightly greased baking sheet, about 2-inches apart, and bake 15 to 20 minutes, until edges are lightly browned. Be careful not to over bake. Let tea cakes rest on baking sheet for 2 minutes before transferring to cooling rack. Refrigerate any leftovers. Makes roughly 18 teacakes.

Chicken

Barbequed Chicken Breasts ~ 77
Chicken and Apricot Curry ~ 77
Chicken Cacciatore ~ 78
Chicken Creole ~ 79
Chicken with Blackberries ~ 80
Chicken with Lentils ~ 81
Chicken with Tomatoes, Potatoes and Olives ~ 82
Curried Chicken and Dumplings ~ 83
Orange Glazed Cornish Hens ~ 84
Roasted Quail with Rosemary ~ 85
Roasted Sausages and Vegetables ~ 85
Safari Chicken ~ 86

Barbequed Chicken Breasts

6 to 8 boneless skinless additive-free chicken breast halves
1/2 barbecue sauce recipe (see recipe)

Preheat oven to 375°F. Place chicken breasts in large flat baking dish. Pour barbeque sauce evenly over chicken. Bake on lower rack in oven for 1 hour or until chicken is cooked through, basting every 15 minutes. If chicken gets too brown, tent loosely with foil. Makes 6 to 8 servings.

Chicken and Apricot Curry

2-1/2 pounds additive-free chicken pieces, skinned
1/2 teaspoon chili powder
1 tablespoon Garam Masala (see recipe)
1 (1-inch) piece fresh ginger, grated
2 cloves garlic, minced
1 cup dried apricots
2/3 cup water
2 tablespoons olive oil
2 onions, finely sliced
1 (14-1/2-ounce) can stewed tomatoes, with juice (or see recipe)
Sea salt to taste
1 tablespoon pure cane sugar
2 tablespoons white wine vinegar

Cut chicken pieces into 4 sections and put in large bowl. Add chili powder, Garam Masala, ginger and garlic. Mix well to coat chicken pieces. Cover and place in refrigerator 2 to 3 hours. While chicken is marinating, combine apricots and water in a small bowl, and soak until chicken is marinated. Heat oil in large saucepan and add chicken pieces. Cook over high heat until browned all over, about 5 minutes. Remove from pan and set aside. Add onions to pan and cook, stirring frequently, about 5 minutes, until soft. Return chicken to pan with tomatoes. Cover and cook over low heat 20 minutes. Drain apricots, add to pan with salt, sugar, and vinegar. Simmer, covered, 10 to 15 minutes, until tender. Serve hot. Makes 4 servings.

Chicken Cacciatore

1 whole additive-free chicken (3 to 4 pounds), cut up
1 cup onion, chopped
1 cup green Bell pepper, chopped
3 cloves garlic, minced
3 tablespoons extra-virgin olive oil
2 (14-1/2-ounce) cans stewed tomatoes (or see recipe)
2 teaspoons oregano
2 teaspoons sea salt
1/2 teaspoon freshly ground black pepper
3 bay leaves
3/4 cup chicken stock (see recipe)
Rice or gluten-free noodles (optional)

Heat oil over medium-high heat in large skillet until it begins to smoke. Working in batches, brown chicken on all sides, stirring frequently, about 10 minutes. Remove chicken and drain excess grease, leaving a tablespoon or two. Add chopped onion, green pepper, and garlic. Sauté until onion is tender. Stir in stewed tomatoes, chicken stock, oregano, salt, pepper and bay leaves. Add chicken and bring to a boil. Reduce heat, cover, and simmer 45 minutes, or until chicken is tender. While chicken is simmering, cook rice or noodles according to directions on package. When chicken is done, discard bay leaves and serve hot. Makes 6 to 8 servings.

Chicken Creole

4 boneless, skinless additive-free chicken breasts, cut into 1-inch
     cubes
2 tablespoons extra-virgin olive oil
1 large onion, coarsely chopped
2 cloves garlic, minced
1 cup mushrooms, coarsely chopped
1 medium green Bell pepper, seeded and coarsely chopped
2 large vine-ripened tomatoes, coarsely chopped
1/2 cup dry white wine
1/4 teaspoon dried red pepper flakes
Fresh parsley, finely chopped, for garnish (optional)

Heat 1 tablespoon oil in large skillet over medium heat. Add
chicken and sauté until chicken turns cream colored on all sides,
about 5 minutes. Transfer to plate and set aside. Add remaining oil
to pan and heat. Add onion and garlic and sauté, stirring
occasionally, until onion is transparent, about 5 minutes. Add Bell
pepper and cook until tender, about 2 to 3 minutes. Add
mushrooms and cook until tender, stirring frequently, about 2
minutes. Add tomatoes, wine and red pepper flakes. Stir well and
bring to a boil. Reduce heat and simmer uncovered to blend flavors,
about 5 minutes. Return chicken to skillet, cover and simmer until
the chicken and vegetables are tender, about 10 minutes. Spoon
into individual bowls and garnish with parsley. Serve while still hot.
Makes 4 servings.

Chicken with Blackberries

1/2 cup dry white wine
1-1/2 pounds boneless additive-free chicken
3 tablespoons fresh thyme
3/4 teaspoons sweet paprika
1/2 cup chicken stock (see recipe)
2 tablespoons pure cane light brown sugar
2 garlic cloves, minced
2 tablespoons white wine vinegar
1 teaspoon extra-virgin olive oil
1/2 cup fresh blackberries

Preheat oven to 375°F. Pour 1/4 of the wine into large baking dish.
Arrange chicken pieces in dish. Sprinkle with thyme, 1/2 teaspoon
of paprika, and season with salt and pepper. Bake 35 minutes,
adding remaining wine and stock to the pan as juices evaporate.
Baste chicken occasionally. In a small bowl, combine brown sugar
with blackberries, garlic, vinegar, oil and the remaining paprika.
Spoon mixture over chicken, and continue cooking about 10
minutes, basting occasionally, until juices run clear when the
chicken is pierced with fork. Transfer chicken to serving platter and
cover loosely with foil. Pour cooking juices into small saucepan and
bring to a boil over medium-high heat. Cook until reduced by half,
about 2 to 3 minutes. Spoon sauce over the chicken. Garnish
chicken with fresh blueberries and serve. Makes 4 servings.

Chicken with Lentils

8-ounces boneless additive-free chicken breasts, cubed
1-1/4 cup red split lentils
3 cups water plus 2/3 cups water
1/2 teaspoon turmeric
4 tablespoons extra-virgin olive oil
6 green cardamom pods, bruised
1 onion, finely sliced
1 (1/2-inch) piece fresh ginger, grated
Sea salt to taste
Cayenne pepper to taste
2 tablespoons lemon juice
1 teaspoon cumin seeds
2 garlic cloves, finely sliced

Wash lentils, place in large saucepan and add 3 cups water and turmeric. Bring to boil, then reduce heat, cover and simmer 20 to 30 minutes, or until cooked. Drain and set aside. Heat half the oil in large saucepan. Add cardamom pods and sauté 1 minute. Add onions and sauté, stirring frequently, about 8 minutes, until golden brown. Add chicken and sauté 5 minutes, until browned all over. Add ginger and sauté 1 minute more. Season with salt and cayenne. Stir in lemon juice and 2/3 cup water. Cover and simmer 25 to 30 minutes, or until chicken is tender. Stir in lentil mixture and cook, stirring, 5 minutes more. Heat remaining oil over medium heat in a small skillet, add cumin seeds and garlic and sauté 1 to 2 minutes, until garlic is golden. Transfer chicken and lentil mixture to serving dish and pour garlic mixture over top. Serve hot. Makes 4 servings.

Chicken with Potatoes, Tomatoes and Olives

1 pound additive-free chicken breasts, cut into 1-1/2-inch chunks
3 cloves garlic, minced
1/4 teaspoon sea salt
2 teaspoons lemon juice
3 tablespoons extra-virgin olive oil
1 lemon, sliced thin (optional)
1 pound small red potatoes, quartered
4 plum tomatoes
10 black brined olives, pitted (see note)
1 tablespoon fresh rosemary

Preheat oven to 400°F. Place potatoes in medium bowl and toss
with garlic, olive oil, salt and lemon juice until coated. Arrange in
large glass baking dish, and cook 20 minutes. Remove from heat.
Add chicken. Sprinkle with olives, tomatoes and rosemary, and
arrange with lemon slices. Reduce heat to 350 °F and cook for 30
minutes, or until chicken and potatoes are cooked through. Discard
lemon slices before serving. Makes 4 servings.

Make sure the olives are brined with white wine vinegar, not
distilled white vinegar, which may contain corn or gluten.

Curried Chicken and Dumplings

1 pound boneless, skinless additive-free chicken breasts, cubed
2 tablespoons extra-virgin olive oil
3 yellow onions, finely chopped
1/2 teaspoon tomato paste
1/4 teaspoon onion powder
1 teaspoon turmeric
1-2 teaspoons red chili powder
1 teaspoon cumin
1 (3-inch) cinnamon stick
1 bay leaf
1/2 teaspoon Garam Masala (see recipe)
2 tablespoons fresh cilantro, chopped, for garnish (optional)
1/2 cup water (divided)
Spinach and Bean Dumplings (optional, see recipe)

Marinade:
1 (1-inch) piece fresh ginger, grated
4 cloves garlic
1/4 cup water

Place chicken cubes in large sealable plastic bag. Blend ginger and garlic with water, and add to chicken. Refrigerate 1 hour. Heat oil over medium heat in heavy skillet, and add onion powder, cinnamon stick and bay leaf. Sauté 3 minutes. Reduce heat to low, add onions and sauté until golden brown, stirring occasionally, about 20 minutes. Add turmeric, red chili pepper, cumin powder and tomato paste. Sauté for 1 minute. Add chicken pieces to onion mixture and combine so all pieces are coated. Add 1/4 cup water and stir well. Cook on medium-low for approximately 15 minutes or until thoroughly cooked. Add Garam Masala when chicken is almost cooked and mix again. Garnish with cilantro serve with Spinach and Bean Dumplings, if desired. Makes 4 servings.

Orange Glazed Cornish Hens

1 cup onion, finely chopped
1 cup celery, finely chopped
3 tablespoons extra-virgin olive oil
3 cups rice of choice, cooked
4 teaspoons pure cane sugar
1 teaspoon sea salt
1/2 teaspoon dried thyme
1/4 cup orange zest
4 (1-1/4 pound) Cornish hens

Glaze:
1 cup orange juice
1/4 cup corn-free honey (see note)
1/4 cup canola oil
1 tablespoon orange zest

Preheat oven to 350°F. In large skillet, sauté onion and celery in oil.
Add cooked rice, sugar, salt, thyme and orange zest, and mix well.
Loosely stuff hens. Place hens breast side up on a rack in a shallow
baking pan. In a small bowl, combine glaze ingredients. Spoon
some over hens. Bake uncovered for 40 minutes, brushing often
with glaze drippings. Cover and bake 40 minutes longer, until juices
run clear, while continuing to brush with glaze. Serve hot on
individual plates. Makes 4 servings.

Always use caution when buying honey. Unless you buy certified
100% pure organic, it may contain unlabeled high fructose corn
syrup. Honey can be replaced with agave nectar in many recipes.

Roasted Quail with Rosemary

8 quail, fresh or thawed
1 package Al Fresco Fresh Sweet Italian Style Chicken Sausages
3 tablespoons sun-dried tomatoes, finely chopped
1 cup dry white wine
1 tablespoon fresh rosemary, chopped
1 clove garlic, minced
Sea salt and freshly ground pepper to taste
Small bunch fresh parsley, chopped, for garnish (optional)

Preheat oven to 375°F. Rinse quail and pat dry. Tuck wing tips under backs. Remove sausage from casing and mix with tomatoes. Put mixture inside quails. Tie legs together with twine, and place in covered casserole. Add wine, rosemary, garlic and salt and pepper to taste. Cover and bake for 1 hour. Uncover and cook, basting several times, for 30 to 40 minutes longer, until quail is tender and browned. Transfer to serving platter and cover to keep warm. Place casserole on top of stove and bring liquid to a simmer over medium heat, stirring constantly. Cook until thickened and reduced. Spoon over quail. Sprinkle with parsley, if desired. Makes 4 to 8 servings.

Roasted Sausages with Vegetables

2 pounds red potatoes, washed, and cut into 1-inch chunks
2 green Bell peppers, cored, seeded, and cut into 1-inch pieces
2 red Bell peppers, cored, seeded, and cut into 1-inch pieces
2 medium onions, cut into 1-inch chunks
1/3 cup extra-virgin olive oil
Sea salt and freshly ground black pepper to taste
1 package Al Fresco Fresh Sweet Italian Style Chicken Sausages

Preheat oven to 450°F. Coat vegetables with oil, and place in single layer on large roasting pan. Sprinkle with salt and pepper to taste. Roast vegetables, stirring once or twice, for 45 minutes. Pierce each sausage several times with a fork. Place sausages on top of vegetables. Bake 15 to 30 minutes, or until sausages and vegetables are cooked through. Serve hot. Makes 8 servings.

Safari Chicken

3 cups additive-free chicken, cooked and cut into small chunks
1 green pepper cut into chunks
1 onion, cut into chunks
1 to 2 tablespoons olive oil
1 can (6-ounces) tomato paste
3/4 cup sunflower seed butter
2-1/2 cups chicken stock (see recipe)
1-1/2 teaspoons sea salt
1 teaspoon chili powder
1 teaspoon pure cane sugar
1/4 teaspoon nutmeg
Cooked white rice (optional)
Banana slices for garnish (optional)

In heavy skillet large enough to hold all ingredients, add oil and heat over medium-high heat. Add pepper and onion, and sauté until browned but just tender, 5 to 8 minutes. Combine tomato paste and sunflower seed butter in medium bowl. Add chicken stock and seasonings, and mix well. Add to skillet with peppers and onions. Stir in cooked chicken. Reduce heat to medium, and cook until heated through and well combined, stirring constantly, about 3 to 5 minutes. Serve over a bed of white rice, if desired. Makes 6 servings.

Dips and Condiments

Apple Butter

10 apples, peeled, cored and cut into quarters
1 cup pure cane dark brown sugar (see note)
1/2 cup of water
1/2 teaspoon cinnamon
1/2 teaspoon nutmeg
1/4 teaspoon allspice
1/4 teaspoon cloves

Place all ingredients in a large saucepan over medium-high heat and cook until tender, stirring occasionally, about apples begin to break down and soften. Reduce heat to medium-low, and continue to simmer until apples thicken and liquid has been reduced by about eighty percent, about 45 minutes. Cool mixture slightly. Blend apples until they are the consistency of a thick apple sauce. They can be mashed with a potato masher as well.
Keeps two weeks in the refrigerator. Freezes well. Makes 3 jars.

Dark brown sugar can be replaced with 1/2 cup white sugar and 2 tablespoons corn-free molasses or Yacon syrup for each 1/2 cup.

Black Bean Dip

1 tablespoon extra-virgin olive oil
3 cloves garlic, coarsely chopped
1 (15-ounce) can black beans, drained and rinsed
1 lime, juiced
1/3 cup fresh cilantro, coarsely chopped
Sea salt to taste

Dipping suggestions:
Rice chips
Fresh veggies

Place ingredients in food processor or blender, and blend until mixture becomes a smooth paste. Serve with dipping suggestion of choice. May be refrigerated up to 1 week. Makes 4 to 6 servings.

Cilantro-Lime Pesto

1 cup pumpkin seeds, shelled
1 cup cilantro, packed
1/2 cup extra-virgin olive oil
1/4 cup lime juice
1 teaspoon sea salt
4 cloves garlic

In large skillet, toast pumpkin seeds over medium heat until puffed, about 4 or 5 minutes. Add all ingredients to food processor, and process until smooth. There will still be small chunks of seeds in the presto. Good on pizza, chicken, and toast. Makes enough for 2 pizza's, 4 whole boneless chicken breasts, or 8 to 12 spread servings, depending on use.

Cranberry Relish

1 (16-ounce) package fresh cranberries
1 medium pear, diced
1 medium apple, diced
1/4 cup corn-free honey (see note)
1 teaspoon horseradish
1 tablespoon balsamic vinegar

Blend cranberries in a blender or food processor. In a bowl, combine blended cranberries and rest of ingredients. Chill, and serve cold. Makes 2-1/2 to 3 cups relish.

Always use caution when buying honey. Unless you buy certified 100% pure organic, it may contain unlabeled high fructose corn syrup. Honey can be replaced with agave nectar in many recipes.

Cranberry Sauce with Apricots

2 (12-ounce) bags fresh cranberries
2/3 cup orange juice (with lots of pulp)
1/2 cup dried apricots, halved and cut in strips
1/2 cup pure cane sugar
1/2 cup pure cane light brown sugar
1 teaspoon orange zest
Pinch of sea salt

In large saucepan over medium-high heat, bring all ingredients to a boil, stirring frequently. Cook, stirring occasionally, until cranberries pop and mixture thickens, about 10 minutes. Cool and serve. Makes 6 to 8 servings.

Ginger Papaya Salsa

1 medium papaya, diced
1 tablespoons cilantro, minced
1 teaspoon fresh ginger, grated
1 tablespoon lime juice

Combine all ingredients in a bowl. Chill, and serve. Makes 2 to 4 servings.

Harissa

10 dried red chili peppers
1 roasted red pepper, diced
4 cloves garlic, minced
1/2 teaspoon salt
1 tablespoon coriander seeds
1 tablespoon caraway seeds
1/2 tablespoon cumin seeds
1/2 teaspoon cinnamon
2 tablespoons extra-virgin olive oil, plus more for top

In heavy skillet over medium-high heat, dry-roast chili peppers 1 to 2 minutes. Remove from heat and add just enough water to cover chilies. Cover and let sit 30 to 45 minutes (or until soft). Remove from water and remove stems and seeds. Be careful not to touch your eyes or face until after you wash your hands thoroughly. In same skillet, toast seeds until fragrant, about 30 to 45 seconds, stirring frequently. Combine spices with remaining ingredients in blender or food processor, and blend to smooth paste. Drizzle in some more oil if too thick. Place in airtight container, drizzle small amount of oil on top, and store in refrigerator. The oil prevents the paste from developing a dry crust. Can also be made with milder chilies. Makes 12 servings.

Harissa is a spicy North African chili paste. It's often used as a condiment, but is also added to spice up meats, stews and sauces.

Hummus

3/4 cup chickpeas, drained (reserve liquid)
3 large lemons, juiced
1/2 cup (4-ounces) tahini
2 cloves garlic, minced
1/4 teaspoon sea salt
2 teaspoons extra-virgin olive oil
Pinch of paprika, for garnish (optional)

In blender or food processor, add chickpeas and process to crumbly
texture, scraping down sides as needed. Add lemon juice, tahini,
garlic and salt and puree until smooth, about 30 seconds. If mixture
is too thick, add reserved chickpea liquid 1 tablespoon at a time
until desired texture is achieved. Scrape dip into small serving bowl.
Place in airtight container, drizzle small amount of oil on top, and
store in refrigerator. The oil prevents the dip from developing a dry
crust. Sprinkle with paprika. Makes 6 servings.

Ketchup

2 (6-ounce) cans tomato paste
1/2 cup apple cider vinegar
5 tablespoons agave nectar
1 teaspoon corn-free molasses (see note)
1 tablespoon garlic powder
1 tablespoon onion powder
1/4 teaspoon ground allspice
1/4 teaspoon ground cloves
1/2 (3-inch) stick cinnamon
1 teaspoon sea salt
2-1/2 cups water

In medium saucepan over medium heat, combine everything and
bring to boil, stirring frequently. Reduce heat to medium-low and
simmer until mixture has reduced to desired consistency, about 40
minutes. Store in airtight container in refrigerator up to 2 weeks.
Makes roughly 2 cups of ketchup, depending on consistency. Note:
Molasses can be replaced with equal amounts of Yacon Syrup.

Mango Chutney

2 mangoes, peeled, seeded and sliced thin
1 red chili, seeded and thinly sliced
1/4 cup raisins
2 tablespoons fresh mint, chopped
Pinch of onion powder
1/2 teaspoon ground cumin
1/4 teaspoon cayenne pepper
1/2 teaspoon ground coriander
Mint sprigs, to garnish

Combine mango slices in medium bowl with chili, raisins and
chopped mint. In separate small bowl, combine onion powder,
cumin, cayenne and coriander. Sprinkle over mango mixture and
stir gently to coat. Cover and refrigerate at least 2 hours before use.
Serve cold, garnished with mint sprigs. Makes about 2 cups.

Mayonnaise Substitute

1/2 cup cold rice milk
1/4 teaspoon prepared yellow mustard
2 teaspoons lemon juice (more to taste)
1/8 teaspoon freshly ground white pepper
1/4 teaspoon guar gum
2 tablespoons extra-virgin olive oil
Medicine dropper (to add the oil)
1/4 teaspoon sea salt

Combine rice milk, mustard, lemon juice and pepper in blender. Blend until well combined. Add guar gum, and blend until foamy. Set blender on high speed. Using a medicine dropper, slowly add oil one drop at a time through hole in lid of blender. It may splatter, so keep a hand ready to cover the hole. The mixture will begin to thicken as you add the oil. Do this very slowly, one drop at a time. If you add the oil too fast, it won't emulsify. Once all the oil has been added, blend until smooth and creamy. Add salt, and adjust lemon juice if desired. Blend to incorporate. Store in refrigerator for up to one week. Makes about 3/4 cup.

Roasted Pear Chutney

6 tablespoons pure cane dark brown sugar (see note)
1 tablespoon lemon juice
1/4 teaspoon ground cinnamon
3 ripe Bosc pears, peeled, cored and quartered
1 cup red onion, chopped
1/2 cup golden raisins
1/4 cup apple cider vinegar
1/4 cup corn-free honey (see note)
1 teaspoon fresh rosemary, minced
1 teaspoon fresh ginger, grated
1/4 teaspoon crushed red pepper

Preheat oven to 400°F. Grease a rimmed baking sheet. In a bowl, whisk together 1 tablespoon brown sugar, lemon juice and cinnamon. Add pears and toss until coated. Arrange pears on baking sheet and roast until tender, about 15 minutes. Cool slightly, and cut into 1/2-inch cubes. In a medium saucepan, bring remaining ingredients to a boil. Reduce heat to medium-low and simmer 5 minutes. Transfer to large bowl. Stir pears into bowl and let cool. Cover and refrigerate until chilled. Goes great with chicken, turkey and pork. Makes 8 to 10 servings.

Dark brown sugar can be replaced with 1/2 cup white sugar and 2 tablespoons corn-free molasses or Yacon syrup for each 1/2 cup.

Always use caution when buying honey. Unless you buy certified 100% pure organic, it may contain unlabeled high fructose corn syrup. Honey can be replaced with agave nectar in many recipes.

Sundried Tomato Hummus

1/4 cup (packed) dry-packed sundried tomatoes
1 (15-ounce) can chickpeas, rinsed and drained
1 teaspoon ground cumin
1 clove garlic
2 tablespoons lemon juice
Large pinch sea salt
1-1/2 tablespoons tahini
2 tablespoons extra-virgin olive oil
1/4 cup water

In small saucepan bring tomatoes and enough water to cover them to a boil. Remove from heat and allow tomatoes to rehydrate 5 to 10 minutes. Drain and place in blender or food processor. Add remaining ingredients and process until smooth, scraping down sides with rubber spatula if necessary. Makes 8 servings.

Sweet Pickle Relish

2 cups finely chopped, seeded cucumber
1/2 cup finely chopped onion
1/2 cup apple cider vinegar
1 teaspoon sea salt, divided
1/4 cup agave nectar
1 teaspoon arrowroot starch / flour, dissolved in 1 teaspoon water

Toss chopped cucumber and onions with 3/4 teaspoon salt and place in strainer over bowl for 3 hours to drain water out. Discard liquid, rinse salt from cucumbers and onions, and squeeze with clean paper towels to draw out as much liquid as possible. In small saucepan, add vinegar, agave nectar and salt and bring to boil over medium heat. Continue to boil until mixture is reduced by half, about 5 minutes. Add cucumber and onion mixture to brine and simmer, stirring occasionally, about 2 minutes. Stir in arrowroot and water mixture, and simmer 1 minute, stirring constantly. Cool and refrigerate. Should keep 1 month in refrigerator. Makes about 2 cups relish.

Can be mixed with Mayonnaise Substitute or Soy Free Vegenaise by Follow Your Heart for homemade Tartar Sauce. See recipes.

Caution: Although the pea protein in Soy Free Vegenaise is not hydrolyzed, it may still contain enough naturally occurring free glutamate to serve as an MSG-trigger in highly sensitive people.

Tartar Sauce

1 cup mayonnaise substitute (see recipe) or Soy Free Vegenaise
1/2 cup corn-free sweet pickle relish (see recipe)
1 teaspoon lemon juice
Sea salt and pepper to taste

Mix all ingredients together in a bowl. Refrigerate until ready to use. Makes 1-1/2 cups. Caution: Although the pea protein in Soy Free Vegenaise is not hydrolyzed, it may still contain enough naturally occurring free glutamate to serve as an MSG-trigger in highly sensitive people.

Watermelon Rind Pickles

8 cups watermelon rind cubes (1 large watermelon)
1/2 cup pickling salt
2 quarts water
2 cups white wine vinegar
3 cups pure cane sugar
1 lemon, thinly sliced
2 (3-inch) cinnamon sticks
1 teaspoon allspice berries
1 teaspoon whole cloves
1/2 cup fresh maraschino cherries, halved and seeds removed (optional)

Remove skin and pink from rind. Cut rind into 1 inch cubes. Soak cubes overnight in brine mixture of pickling salt and water. The next day, drain and rinse. Drain again. Add more fresh water to cover, and simmer until tender. Drain. Make syrup of vinegar, sugar, lemon, and spices tied in a cheesecloth bag. Simmer 5 minutes. Add rind and cook until clear. If using cherries, combine with rind mixture and simmer 2 more minutes. Let cool, and store in clean glass jars in refrigerator. Allow to set at least two weeks before eating. Makes 4 pints.

Dressings, Sauces and Seasonings

Baby Back Rib Rub

1 tablespoon cumin
1 tablespoon thyme
1 teaspoon sea salt
1-1/2 teaspoons freshly ground black pepper
1/2 teaspoon ground cayenne
1 teaspoon garlic powder

Combine all ingredients in small bowl. Store in airtight container until ready for use. Makes just under 1/4 cup of rub mix.

Since this rub keeps well, you might want to double the recipe to keep more on hand ready to use. Caution: Do *not* reuse extra rub after it has been in contact with meat.

Balsamic Blueberry Pan Sauce

1 tablespoon extra-virgin olive oil
1 large shallot, thinly sliced
1/4 teaspoon sea salt
Pinch of freshly ground black pepper
Pinch of oregano
1 cup fresh blueberries
1/4 cup water
1 tablespoon balsamic vinegar

Heat oil in a small saucepan over medium low heat. Add shallot and sauté until tender, about 3 to 4 minutes. Stir in salt, pepper and oregano. Add blueberries, water and vinegar. Using a potato masher or a fork, gently mash blueberries, leaving a few chunky pieces. Cook sauce for 3 to 5 minutes, stirring often, until thickly bubbling and purplish-blue. Serve warm with chicken or turkey, or whole grain pilafs. May be refrigerated and reheated before serving. Makes about 1 cup of sauce.

Barbeque Sauce

2 tablespoons extra-virgin olive oil
2 tablespoons onion, finely chopped
1 tablespoon green Bell pepper
1 cup water
1 cup additive-free ketchup (see recipe)
1 teaspoon sea salt
1 teaspoon celery seed
2 tablespoons pure cane dark brown sugar (see note)
2 teaspoons lemon juice
2 teaspoons dry mustard

Heat oil in medium saucepan over medium high heat. Cook onion and peppers until tender. Add remaining ingredients. Bring to a boil, then reduce heat and simmer 20 to 30 minutes. Remove from heat and let cool. Makes about 2-1/2 cups.

Dark brown sugar can be replaced with 1/2 cup white sugar and 2 tablespoons corn-free molasses or Yacon syrup for each 1/2 cup.

Cranberry Vinaigrette

1/4 cup dried cranberries
1/4 cup hot water
1/4 cup orange juice
1 tablespoon red wine vinegar
1 teaspoon prepared yellow mustard
1/4 cup canola oil

Salad suggestion:
Mixed salad greens
1 pear, thinly sliced
4 fresh mandarin oranges, peeled, seeded and membrane removed
1/2 cup dried cranberries

Rehydrate cranberries by placing them in hot water in small bowl. Set aside 30 minutes, then drain. In food processor or blender, puree cranberries with orange juice. Add vinegar and mustard. Blend to combine. Gradually add canola oil while still blending until thickened slightly. Chill until ready to serve. Makes about 1/2 cup.

For the salad: Toss the salad ingredients in a large bowl. Mix dressing into the salad, or serve on the side.

Garam Masala

1 tablespoon plus 1 teaspoon cardamom seeds
2 (3-inch) cinnamon sticks, crushed
2 teaspoons whole cloves
1 tablespoon plus 1 teaspoon black peppercorns
3 tablespoons cumin seeds
3 tablespoons coriander seeds

Put all spices in a heavy skillet and dry roast over medium heat 5 to 10 minutes, until browned, stirring constantly. Cool completely then grind to a fine powder in a coffee grinder, or with a mortar and pestle. Store in an airtight jar up to 2 months. Makes about 1/2 cup.

General Purpose Rub

1/4 cup sea salt
4 tablespoons freshly ground black pepper
2 tablespoons freshly ground white pepper
1-1/2 teaspoons cayenne pepper
2 tablespoons onion powder
1-1/2 teaspoons ground cumin
4 tablespoons garlic powder
2 tablespoons hot paprika

Combine well, and store in a sealed container in a cool, dry place. When ready to use, apply rub thoroughly and evenly. After applying, cover meat with plastic wrap or aluminum foil and refrigerate. This allows flavors to penetrate meat. Large cuts of meat can sit overnight or for several days. Makes about 1 cup of rub.

Do not re-use extra rub after it has been in contact with meat.

Italian Dressing

2/3 cup canola oil
1/3 cup apple cider vinegar
1/4 teaspoon dry mustard
1/4 teaspoon garlic powder
1/8 teaspoon freshly ground black pepper
1/4 teaspoon pure cane sugar
3 tablespoons lemon juice
1/4 teaspoon basil
1/8 teaspoon oregano

Place all ingredients in a tightly sealed jar and shake well. Keeps well in refrigerator. Makes just over 1 cup of dressing.

Memphis Rub

1/4 cup paprika
1 tablespoon pure cane sugar
1 tablespoon pure cane dark brown sugar (see note)
2 teaspoons sea salt
1 teaspoon celery salt
1 teaspoon freshly ground black pepper
1 teaspoon cayenne pepper (more to taste)
1 teaspoon dry mustard
1 teaspoon garlic powder
1 teaspoon onion powder

Combine well, and store in a sealed container in a cool, dry place. When ready to use, apply rub thoroughly and evenly. Cover the meat with plastic wrap or aluminum foil and refrigerate. This allows the flavors to really penetrate the meat. Large cuts of meat can sit overnight or for several days. I prefer mine more heavily rubbed, so I usually double the recipe. Makes about 1/2 cup.

Dark brown sugar can be replaced with 1/2 cup white sugar and 2 tablespoons corn-free molasses or Yacon syrup for each 1/2 cup. Do not reuse extra rub after it has been in contact with meat.

Russian Dressing

1/4 cup agave nectar
2/3 cup canola oil
1/3 cup apple cider vinegar
1/4 teaspoon dry mustard
1/8 teaspoon garlic powder
1/8 teaspoon pepper
1/2 cup additive-free ketchup (see recipe)
1/4 teaspoon chili powder
1/8 teaspoon onion powder
1 tablespoon Worcestershire sauce substitute (optional, see recipe)

Place all ingredients in a jar. Tightly seal it, and shake well. Keeps well in the refrigerator. Makes just over 2 cups of dressing.

Seasoned Salt

2 teaspoons freshly ground black pepper
1 teaspoon onion salt
1 teaspoon onion powder
1 teaspoon garlic salt
1 teaspoon garlic powder
1 teaspoon ground cumin
1 teaspoon dried marjoram
1 teaspoon dried parsley
1/2 teaspoon curry powder
1/4 cup sea salt

Combine well, and store in a sealed container in a cool, dry place until ready for use. Makes about 1/2 cup.

Sesame Ginger Dressing

6 tablespoons cold-pressed sesame oil
2 tablespoons Coconut Aminos (see note)
1 tablespoon agave nectar
1 tablespoon sesame seeds
1 clove garlic, minced
1/2 teaspoon fresh ginger, grated
1/2 teaspoon lime zest
1/4 teaspoon crushed chili pepper

In small bowl, whisk all ingredients together until combined. Great on salads, or as a dipping sauce for fresh spring rolls. Makes 1/2 cup.

Coconut Aminos can be substituted for soy sauce in dressings, marinades and other recipes. This product is not derived from the nut of the coconut tree.

Southern Barbeque Rub

1/4 cup pure cane light brown sugar
2 tablespoons sea salt
1/4 cup freshly ground black pepper
1/4 cup hot paprika
1 teaspoon dry mustard
1 tablespoon onion powder
2 tablespoons garlic powder
1 teaspoon ground cayenne (more to taste)

Combine well, and store in a sealed container in a cool, dry place. When ready to use, apply rub thoroughly and evenly. After applying, cover meat with plastic wrap or aluminum foil and refrigerate. This allows flavors to penetrate meat. Large cuts of meat can sit overnight or for several days. Makes about 1 cup.

Do not reuse extra rub after it has been in contact with meat.

Soy Sauce Substitute

2 cups beef stock (see recipe)
1/4 cup apple cider vinegar
2 teaspoons corn-free molasses (see note)
1/8 teaspoon ground ginger
Pinch of freshly ground black pepper
Pinch of garlic powder

Place all ingredients in saucepan over medium-high heat. Whisk until combined. Reduce heat to medium-low, and simmer until reduced by at least half. Store in refrigerator for up to 1 month. Makes about 1 cup.

This is a good recipe to make in large batches and store for later use in main dishes, soups, stews, etc. A neat trick is to use plastic ice-cube trays, and pour 2 tablespoons into each section. Once frozen, pop them out into a sealable plastic bag, and mark the contents.

Molasses can be replaced with equal amounts of Yacon Syrup.

Spaghetti Sauce

4 tablespoons extra-virgin olive oil, more if needed
4 cloves garlic, minced
2 pounds ground pork
1 pound ground sirloin
1 (32-ounce) can tomato paste
1 teaspoon pure cane sugar
2 tablespoons sea salt
1 teaspoon freshly ground black pepper
6 large or 8 medium ripe tomatoes, peeled, seeded and diced
1 teaspoons thyme
1 teaspoons oregano

To skin tomatoes, hold on slotted spoon in pot of rapidly boiling water until skin starts to crack and pull away from tomato, about 1 minute or so. Remove, let cool, and discard skins. Slice and remove seeds. Heat oil in large, heavy skillet over medium-high heat. Add pork and sirloin and cook, stirring frequently until browned and cooked, about 10 to 15 minutes. Break up larger chunks of meat while cooking. Add tomato paste and cook 10 to 15 minutes, stirring frequently. Add tomatoes and seasonings. Bring to a boil, then reduce heat and simmer partially covered 2 to 4 hours. If mixing with gluten-free pasta, reserve a little pasta water, then mix with sauce. Top pasta with a little more sauce. Freezes well.

Spicy Asian Dipping Sauce

2 tablespoons apple cider vinegar
1 teaspoon lime juice
1 teaspoon Coconut Aminos (see note)
1 tablespoon water
2-1/2 teaspoons agave nectar
1/2 teaspoon lime zest
1 clove garlic, minced
1 chili pepper, seeded, stem removed and minced
1/4 teaspoon sea salt

In small bowl, whisk lime zest and minced garlic together with rest of ingredients. Can be used as a dressing, dipping sauce or marinade. Keeps several weeks in refrigerator. Makes 1/3 cup.

Coconut Aminos can be substituted for soy sauce in dressings, marinades and other recipes. This product is not derived from the nut of the coconut tree.

Teriyaki Marinade and Sauce

1 cup Coconut Aminos (see note)
2 tablespoons white wine vinegar
1 teaspoon dry mustard
1/2 teaspoon garlic powder
1 cup orange juice or water
3 tablespoons pure cane light brown sugar
1 teaspoon fresh ginger, grated
1 teaspoon ground cayenne
1 tablespoon extra-virgin olive oil (for marinade)

Whisk all ingredients except for olive oil together in medium saucepan. Bring to a boil, reduce heat, and stir to combine flavors. For marinade, add 1 tablespoon of olive oil. Makes about 2-1/2 cups.

This is a good recipe to make ahead of time and store for later use. One of the easiest ways to do this is to get some plastic ice-cube trays, and measure out 2 tablespoons into each section. Once frozen, pop them out into a sealable plastic bag, and mark the contents. You now have pre-measured cubes ready to use!

Coconut Aminos can be substituted for soy sauce in dressings, marinades and other recipes. This product is not derived from the nut of the coconut tree.

Thousand Island Dressing

1 cup mayonnaise substitute (see recipe) or Soy Free Vegenaise
1/4 cup additive-free ketchup (see recipe)
2 tablespoon apple cider vinegar
4 teaspoons agave nectar
1/4 cup corn-free sweet pickle relish, drained (see recipe)
2 teaspoons white onion, finely minced
1/4 teaspoon sea salt
1/8 teaspoon freshly ground black pepper

Combine all ingredients except for relish in blender or food processor, and blend well to combine. Transfer to a small bowl. Add relish and mix to combine. Makes about 1-1/2 cups.

Caution: Although the pea protein in Soy Free Vegenaise is not hydrolyzed, it may still contain enough naturally occurring free glutamate to serve as an MSG-trigger in highly sensitive people.

Turkey Gravy

4 cups turkey stock (see recipe)
4 tablespoons turkey fat or extra-virgin olive oil
3-1/3 tablespoons potato starch
2 bay leaves
4 dried porcini mushrooms
2 tablespoons Madeira wine
Sea salt to taste
2 teaspoons potato starch for each 1 cup stock

Bring 4 cups turkey stock to a boil in a medium saucepan. Reduce heat to medium-low. Add bay leaves, mushrooms and wine. Let simmer until reduced to desired concentration. The flavor intensifies the more it reduces. Remove herbs and mushrooms with a slotted spoon. For each cup of turkey stock you wind up with after reducing, you will need 2 teaspoons potato starch. Whisk the starch in a small bowl with enough cold water to make a thin gruel. Mix into stock, whisking constantly. Turn off heat immediately, and remove from heat source. Continue to whisk until gravy thickens, another minute or two. Repeat gruel process with more potato starch if you desire a thicker gravy. Season with salt and serve. Makes 8 to 10 servings.

Turkey Mushroom Gravy

6 tablespoons extra-virgin olive oil
2 shallots, finely chopped
1 pound mixed mushrooms, trimmed and sliced
1/3 cup dry white wine or sherry
4 cups turkey stock (see recipe)
3 tablespoons finely chopped parsley
3 tablespoons potato starch
Sea salt and freshly ground pepper to taste

Heat 3 tablespoons oil in large skillet over medium-high heat. Add shallots and cook, stirring often, until softened, about 5 minutes. Add half of mushrooms to pan, stirring occasionally, until golden, about 5 minutes. Transfer to plate. Repeat with remaining 3 tablespoons oil and mushrooms. Return first batch of mushrooms to pan. Stir in wine or sherry and cook, stirring occasionally, until almost evaporated. Stir in turkey stock and bring to boil, stirring constantly. Shut off heat and remove from heat source. Whisk potato starch in small bowl with enough cold water to make a thin gruel. Mix into stock, whisking constantly. Continue to whisk until gravy thickens, another minute or two. Repeat gruel process with more potato starch if thicker gravy is desired. Season with salt and pepper to taste. Stir in parsley. Keep warm until ready to serve. Makes about 4-1/2 cups.

Worcestershire Sauce Substitute

2 cups apple cider vinegar
1/2 cup corn-free molasses or Yacon syrup
1/2 cup Coconut Aminos (see note)
3 tablespoons mustard seeds
3 tablespoons sea salt
1 tablespoon whole black peppercorns
1 teaspoon whole cloves
1/2 teaspoon curry powder
5 cardamom pods, smashed
1/2 teaspoons crushed red pepper flakes
2 cloves garlic, minced
1 (1-inch) stick cinnamon
1 medium yellow onion, chopped
1 (1/2-inch) piece of ginger, peeled and crushed
1/2 cup agave nectar (add last)

Add only *one* of the following:
1/4 cup tamarind concentrate (paste)
1/4 cup unripe, green mango (peeled) plus 2 tablespoons lemon
    juice, process in food processor into small chunks
1/4 cup dried apricots (read label carefully) plus 2 tablespoons
    lemon juice, process in food processor into small chunks

Combine all ingredients in top list except for agave nectar in
medium saucepan. Add either tamarind concentrate, mango and
lemon pulp, or dried apricot and lemon pulp, and stir. Bring to a
boil, reduce heat to barely a simmer, and cook 15 minutes,
uncovered, stirring occasionally. Add agave nectar and whisk to
combine. Simmer another 5 minutes. Remove from heat and let
cool. Transfer sauce to glass jar with a tight-fitting lid. Refrigerate
for 1 week. Strain to remove solids, and return to jar. Refrigerate up
to 8 months. Makes between 1-1/2 to 2 cups, depending on
evaporation during cooking and how well you strain it.

Coconut Aminos can be substituted for soy sauce in dressings,
marinades and other recipes. This product is not derived from the
nut of the coconut tree.

Frostings, Syrups and Glazes

Blackberry Maple Syrup

1/2 cup maple syrup
1 (12-ounce) package frozen blackberries, thawed
1 teaspoon lemon zest
2 teaspoons lemon juice
1 teaspoon arrowroot starch / flour

Gently mash berries with potato masher, leaving a mix of whole berries, partly broken berries and crushed berries. Stir in maple syrup, and then add berries. Bring mixture to gentle simmer and for 2 to 3 minutes. Remove from heat. In a small bowl, mix arrowroot with equal amount of cold water, then whisk into sauce for about 30 seconds, until mixture thickens. For a thicker sauce, add more arrowroot mixed with water 1 teaspoon at a time until you reach your desired consistency. Cool to desired temperature and serve. Makes 2 cups.

Blueberry Sauce

1 cup fresh or frozen blueberries
1/4 cup water
1/2 cup pulpy orange juice
3/8 cup pure cane sugar
2 teaspoons arrowroot starch / flour
1 teaspoon ground cinnamon

In a saucepan over medium heat, combine blueberries, water, orange juice and sugar. Stir gently until it comes to a boil, taking care not to mash the berries. Remove from heat. In a small bowl, mix arrowroot with equal amount of cold water, then blend into sauce for about 30 seconds, until mixture thickens. For a thicker sauce, add more arrowroot mixed with water 1 teaspoon at a time until you reach your desired consistency. Stir in cinnamon. Goes great with pancakes, waffles, and even broiled chicken breasts! Makes about 2 cups.

Chocolate Maple Cookie Glaze

1/2 cup maple syrup
1 cup dairy-free cocoa powder
2 tablespoons Spectrum brand palm oil shortening, melted
1 teaspoon sea salt
1 teaspoon corn-free vanilla

Combine all ingredients in a blender and process until smooth. Drizzle over cookies, and let set until dry. Makes about 1-1/2 cups of glaze.

Cinnamon Pancake Syrup

1/2 cup agave nectar
1 teaspoon ground cinnamon
Pinch of sea salt

Combine syrup ingredients in a small, heavy bottom saucepan and heat until bubbles start to form around edges of the pan. Do not boil. Let cool to desired temperature, and serve with your favorite pancakes or waffles. Makes 1/2 cup.

Sugar Cookie Frosting

4 cups corn-free powdered sugar (see note)
1/3 cup Spectrum brand palm oil shortening
4 tablespoons rice milk
1 teaspoon corn-free vanilla
Food coloring (optional, read label carefully)

In large bowl, blend sugar and shortening until creamy. Mix in rice milk and vanilla, and combine well. If desired, add food coloring one drop at a time, and mix well to incorporate, until desired color is reached. Makes 3 cups.

Powdered sugar generally contains cornstarch. To make your own, add 1 tablespoon potato starch to 1 cup of sugar and blend in a coffee grinder until you get a fine texture.

Frosting for One

1/4 cup corn-free powdered sugar (see note)
1 tablespoon Spectrum brand palm oil shortening
3/4 teaspoon rice milk
1/8 teaspoon corn-free vanilla

Beat until fluffy. Makes enough for one cupcake or cookie, or one slice of carrot cake.

Powdered sugar generally contains cornstarch. To make your own, add 1 tablespoon potato starch to 1 cup of sugar and blend in a coffee grinder until you get a fine texture.

Whipped Cream Frosting

1/4 cup rice flour
1 cup rice milk
1 cup pure cane sugar
3/4 cup Spectrum brand palm oil shortening
3 tablespoons grape seed oil
1 teaspoon corn-free vanilla
3 tablespoons dairy-free cocoa powder (optional)

In medium saucepan, whisk together rice flour and rice milk until combined. Cook over medium heat, stirring frequently. As mixture begins to thicken, continue to whisk until it reaches the consistency of pudding. Remove from heat and set aside to cool. In a medium mixing bowl, blend shortening and grape seed oil together with electric mixer until smooth, 3 to 4 minutes. Add sugar and blend well. Add vanilla, and cooled flour and milk mixture. Beat another 4 minutes or so, until completely combined. Add cocoa powder if desired, and mix until blended in until completely combined. Frost cake or cupcakes immediately, and refrigerate until ready to serve. Makes about 2 cups.

Lamb

Apricot Lamb Tagine

3/4 cup chickpeas
4 cloves garlic, minced
1 (3-inch) cinnamon stick, broken in half
2 tablespoons extra-virgin olive oil (more if needed)
3 pounds additive-free lamb shoulder, cut into 1-inch cubes
Sea salt and freshly ground black pepper
1 large onion, diced
1/2 teaspoon red pepper flakes
1-1/2 teaspoons ground cinnamon
1 teaspoon paprika
1/2 teaspoon ground cardamom
1 teaspoon dried ginger
1/2 teaspoon turmeric
1 cup stewed tomatoes, with juice (see recipe)
2-1/2 cups chicken stock (see recipe)
1/2 cup dried apricots, cut in half
Cooked couscous
Fresh cilantro, chopped, for garnish (optional)

Heat oil in large heavy skillet over medium-high heat until it begins to smoke. Season lamb with salt and pepper. Working in batches, brown lamb on all sides in oil, about 4 to 7 minutes per batch. Add onion to skillet, reduce heat to medium, season with more salt and pepper, and sauté until tender and begins to turn brown, about 5 to 7 minutes. Add garlic, red pepper flakes, cinnamon, paprika, cardamom, ginger and turmeric. Stir to mix well. Add stewed tomatoes and lamb with any accumulated juices. Bring to a boil. Add stock and return to a boil. Reduce heat to low and partially cover. Simmer, stirring occasionally, until lamb is tender, about 1-1/2 hours. When lamb is about half-way done, prepare couscous according to directions on package and set aside covered to keep warm. When lamb is tender, stir in chickpeas and apricots. Simmer about 5 to 10 more minutes, until apricots are softened. Spoon couscous onto a large, shallow platter, forming a well in center. Spoon lamb in center. Garnish with cilantro if desired. Makes 6 to 8 servings.

Braised Lamb with Mint

2 pounds additive-free lamb shoulder, cut into cubes
1 teaspoon sea salt
1/2 teaspoon freshly ground black pepper
2 tablespoons extra-virgin olive oil (more if needed)
2 cups onion, chopped
6 garlic cloves, chopped
3/4 cup dry red wine
1/2 cup water
2 cups additive-free tomato juice
1 cup chicken stock (see recipe)
1 teaspoon ground cumin
1/2 teaspoon hot Hungarian paprika
3/4 cup carrot, chopped
2 tablespoons fresh parsley, chopped
2 tablespoons peas
1 tablespoon fresh mint, chopped

Season lamb with salt and pepper. Heat oil in large skillet over medium heat until it begins to smoke. Working in batches, cook lamb until brown on all sides, about 4 to 7 minutes per batch, adding more oil if needed. Using a slotted spoon, transfer browned lamb to medium bowl and set aside. Add onions to same skillet and cook over medium heat, stirring occasionally, until softened and light brown, about 5 minutes. Add garlic and cook, stirring constantly, about 1 minute. Add wine and lamb along with any accumulated juices. Simmer lamb until liquid is reduced by half, about 5 minutes. Stir in tomato juice, chicken stock, cumin, paprika and water, and bring to boil. Cover, reduce heat to medium-low, and simmer, stirring occasionally, until lamb is tender and sauce thickens, about 1-1/2 hours. Add chopped carrot and cook, uncovered, stirring occasionally, until carrot is tender, about 15 minutes. Stir in parsley. Transfer braised lamb to a large bowl. Garnish with peas and mint. Makes 4 to 6 servings.

Lamb Curry

1 pound additive-free lamb, cut into 1-inch cubes
1/4 cup extra-virgin olive oil
1 teaspoon turmeric
2 teaspoons red chili powder
1 teaspoon coriander
1 teaspoon Garam Masala (see recipe)
2 onions, finely chopped
2 carrots, chopped
1 (14-1/2 ounce) can stewed tomatoes, with juice (or see recipe)
1 teaspoon sea salt
3 bay leaves
2 cups water
2 teaspoons fresh cilantro (optional)
Basmati rice, cooked

Masala marinade:
4 cloves garlic, minced
1/2 inch piece of ginger, grated
1 green chili, finely chopped

Mix marinade ingredients in medium bowl. Add meat, chili powder, coriander, Garam Masala and salt. Mix well, and let marinate in refrigerator 1 hour. Heat oil in medium saucepan over low heat. Add bay leaves and onions. Sauté until golden brown, about 10 minutes. Add tomatoes and 1/4 cup water. Cover and cook 5 minutes. Add meat and sauté 5 minutes. Add remainder of water slowly and stir. Reduce heat, cover and simmer 2 hours, or until meat is tender. When lamb is almost done, cook basmati rice according to package directions. Add salt to taste. Garnish with cilantro if desired. Serve with rice. Makes 2 to 4 servings.

Lamb in Dill Sauce

2 large potatoes, cut into 1-inch cubes
1/2 cup chopped onion
1-1/2 teaspoons sea salt
1/2 teaspoon freshly ground black pepper
4 sprigs fresh dill, or 1/2 teaspoon dry dill weed
1 bay leaf
2 pounds lean additive-free lamb stew meat, cut into 1-inch cubes
1 cup plus 3 tablespoons water, divided
1 tablespoon potato starch
1 teaspoon pure cane sugar
2 tablespoons lemon juice
Fresh dill for garnish (optional)

Place potatoes in the bottom of a slow cooker, followed by onion, salt, pepper, dill, bay leaf, lamb and 1 cup water. Cover and cook on low 6 to 8 hours. Remove lamb and potatoes with slotted spoon. Cover and keep warm. Discard bay leaf. Turn heat to high. Stir potato starch and remaining 3 tablespoons water in small bowl until smooth. Add half of cooking juices, lemon juice and sugar. Mix well and return to slow cooker. Stir until thickened, should take just a few minutes. Return lamb and potatoes to slow cooker. Cover and cook until heated through, 5 minutes or so. Serve hot, garnished with fresh dill if desired. Makes 6 servings.

Lamb Shish-Kebab

8 metal skewers, at least 10-inches long
1-1/2 pounds additive-free leg of lamb, boned and trimmed of fat
1/4 cup dry white wine
1 lemon, juice and lemon zest reserved
1 tablespoon extra-virgin olive oil
8 bay leaves
2 tablespoons oregano, finely chopped
3 cloves garlic, minced
1/4 teaspoon freshly ground black pepper
Oregano sprigs for garnish (optional)
Lemon wedges for serving (optional)

Cut lamb into 1-inch cubes. Combine wine, lemon zest and juice, oil, bay leaves, oregano and garlic in shallow glass dish and mix well. Add lamb to marinade and stir until lamb is evenly coated. Cover and marinate in refrigerator 2 hours, stirring several times to coat meat. Preheat broiler on high heat and place rack so broiler pan is 3 to 5 inches from heat source. Put lamb evenly on skewers, with 1 bay leaf each. Place lamb on broiler rack and broil until slightly browned, about 2 minutes per side. Reduce heat to medium, brush marinade on lamb and broil 3 more minutes on each side. Brush lamb with marinade one more time and broil until cooked through, about 2 minutes longer per side. To test for doneness, cut a piece of lamb in half. It should be brownish pink inside. Transfer to serving platter, garnish with oregano sprigs and serve with lemon wedges if desired. Makes 4 servings.

Lamb with Onions

1-1/2 pounds additive-free lamb shoulder
1 teaspoon turmeric
1 teaspoon cumin
1 teaspoon coriander
1 (1-inch) piece fresh ginger, grated
2 cloves garlic, minced
3 tablespoons extra-virgin olive oil
1 tablespoon pure cane sugar
4 large onions, sliced into thin rings
1 pound potatoes, peeled and cut into large chunks
1 cup water
Sea salt and cayenne pepper to taste
1 teaspoon Garam Masala (see recipe)
Rosemary sprigs, to garnish (optional)

Trip excess fat from lamb and cut into 1-1/2-inch cubes. Put lamb in glass bowl. Sprinkle with turmeric, cumin, coriander, gingerroot and garlic and stir well. Cover and refrigerate 2 to 3 hours. Heat oil in a heavy saucepan until smoking. Stir in sugar, then add onions and cook over medium high heat 10 minutes, until rich and brown, stirring frequently. Remove onions with a slotted spoon and set aside. Add lamb and cook until browned on all sides. Add potatoes and cook 2 minutes, stirring constantly. Return onions to pan. Add water, salt and cayenne. Bring to boil. Reduce heat, cover and simmer 1-1/2 hours, or until lamb is tender, stirring occasionally. Stir in Garam Masala and serve hot. Garnish with rosemary sprigs if desired. Makes 4 servings.

Roast Leg of Lamb

3 to 4 pounds additive-free leg of lamb, boned and trimmed
8 cloves garlic, minced
3 tablespoons rosemary, chopped
1/4 cup lemon juice
2 teaspoons sea salt
1 teaspoon freshly ground black pepper
3 carrots, peeled and sliced thin
2 onions, quartered then cut into chunks
1-1/2 cups celery, chopped thin

Arrange lamb in glass baking dish. Mix garlic and rosemary. Rub lamb with mixture, making sure to get into the crevices. Pour lemon juice on top and sprinkle with salt. Cover and refrigerate overnight. Preheat oven to 425°F. Cut vegetables and place around lamb. Sprinkle with pepper. Roast lamb and vegetables 15 minutes, then reduce heat to 350°F. After about 20 minutes, check internal temperature with meat thermometer. Continue to check every 5 minutes until temperature reaches 130°F for medium rare. Remove and let rest before carving. Serve with vegetables and pan juices. If vegetables aren't tender yet, place into pan with roasting juice and simmer over medium heat while lamb rests. Makes 6 servings.

Rosemary Lamb Chops

12 additive-free lamb chops
6 tablespoons lemon juice
3 tablespoons fresh rosemary, chopped
3 cloves garlic, minced
1/4 teaspoon sea salt
1/4 teaspoon freshly ground black pepper

Mix lemon juice, rosemary, garlic, salt, and pepper together in small bowl. Rub lamb with mixture. Set aside on plate. Preheat broiler on high heat, and place a heavy oven-safe roasting pan bout 5 to 7 inches under heat source for about 10 minutes to get hot. Once pan is hot, arrange lamb chops in pan and return to broiler. Cook about 4 to 5 minutes, depending on thickness of lamb. Makes 4 servings.

Spiced Lamb Soup

4 ounces split black-eyes peas, soaked overnight
1-1/2 pounds additive-free lamb shoulder, cut into medium sized
    chunks
1/2 teaspoon dried thyme
2 bay leaves
5 cups beef stock (see recipe)
I onion, sliced
8 ounces pumpkin, diced (can substitute butternut squash)
2 cardamom pods
1-1/2 teaspoons turmeric
1 tablespoon chopped, fresh cilantro
1 fresh green chili, seeded and chopped
2 green bananas, cut into medium slices
2 carrots, cut into thin slices
Sea salt and freshly ground black pepper to taste
Shredded carrot for garnish (optional)

Drain peas, place them in saucepan and cover with just enough cold
water to barely cover them. Bring to a boil and boil rapidly for 10
minutes. Reduce heat and simmer, covered, 40 to 50 minutes until
tender, adding more water if necessary. Remove from heat and set
aside to cool. Put lamb in large saucepan, add thyme, bay leaves and
stock or water and bring to a boil. Cover and simmer over medium-
low heat for 1 hour, or until tender. Add onions, pumpkin,
cardamom, turmeric, cilantro, chili, salt and pepper and stir. Bring
back to a simmer and cook uncovered 15 minutes, stirring
occasionally, until pumpkin is tender. When peas are cool, place in a
blender or food processor with their liquid and blend to a smooth
puree. Stir bananas, carrots and pea puree into the soup and cook
10 to 12 minutes, until vegetables are tender. Garnish with shredded
carrot if desired, and serve hot. Makes 4 servings.

Pork

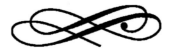

Baby Back Ribs ~ 129
Garlic Pork with Greens ~ 130
Ginger Pork ~ 131
Pulled Pork ~ 132
Roast Pork Shoulder ~ 133
Roast Pork Tenderloin ~ 133
Spice Rubbed Pork Tenderloin ~ 134
Wild Rice Stuffed Pork Chops ~ 135

Baby Back Ribs

2 slabs additive-free baby back ribs
1 cup dry rub mix of choice (see recipes)
1-1/4 cups barbeque sauce (recipe)

Day before you cook the ribs: Carefully remove and discard
membrane and flap of skin from underside of ribs. It helps to slide
a sharp knife underneath to lift up a section, and use a piece of dry
paper-towel to keep a firm grasp as you pull. Pat ribs dry with a
paper towel. Prepare a heavy piece of aluminum foil for each rack,
large enough to set the rack on top, and then wrap around and
cover. Set one rack of ribs on each piece of foil, bottom side up.
Press rub mix well into the bottom of each rack, then turn over and
do the same for the tops. Be sure to get all the edges and crevices.
Seal the foil tightly and refrigerate for 8 to 24 hours. Preheat oven
to 250°F. Remove sealed rib packets from refrigerator and place
them on a baking pan or cookie sheet. Bake in preheated oven for 1
hour. Remove, and with oven mitts on, carefully open one end and
drain out fat. Seal opening, return to oven, and bake for 1 hour.
Repeat fat draining process. Seal opening, and return to oven for 1-
1/2 more hours. Remove ribs from oven. Let rest for 10 minutes,
remove foil and drain any last accumulated liquid. Spread both sides
of ribs with barbecue sauce, return to oven and bake, uncovered for
an additional 30 minutes. Serve hot, with additional sauce if desired.
Makes 4 to 6 servings.

These freeze very well if you prefer to make extra for another time.
I like to pre-slice them, coat with extra barbeque sauce, and store
them in sealable plastic bags. To re-heat, wrap thawed ribs tightly in
foil and bake in preheated 350°F oven for 30 minutes, or until
desired temperature.

Garlic Pork with Greens

2-1/2 pounds additive-free boneless pork shoulder, cut into 1-1/2-
    inch cubes
Sea salt and freshly ground black pepper to taste
2 tablespoons extra-virgin olive oil (more if needed)
1 large yellow onion, finely chopped
2 sprigs fresh thyme
15 to 20 cloves garlic
1 teaspoon fresh rosemary, minced (optional)
2/3 cup dry white wine
1 tablespoon red wine vinegar
2/3 cup beef stock or chicken stock (see recipes)
1-1/4 pound kale, stems removed and leaves cut into strips
White rice, cooked

Season cubed pork generously with salt and pepper. Heat 1
tablespoon olive oil in heavy skillet over medium-high heat. Brown
pork in batches, until well browned on all sides, 6 to 7 minutes
total. Add more oil as needed. Set aside to drain. When finished,
pour off most of oil from pan and return to medium-high heat.
Add onion and thyme and sauté until onion is golden brown, about
5 minutes. Add garlic and rosemary and cook 2 minutes more. Pour
in wine and vinegar and stir to scrape up browned bits from bottom
of skillet. Transfer contents of pan to slow cooker. Add pork and
stock. Stir to combine. Cover and cook on low 5 to 6 hours, stirring
2 to 3 times during first half of cooking time. Stir in kale, re-cover
and cook 1 hour more. The pork and kale should be very tender.
Using a slotted spoon, divide pork and kale among warmed
individual plates. Add scoop of white rice to each plate. Scoop and
discard fat from braising liquid, then drizzle some of the de-fatted
liquid over the rice and meat. Serve immediately. Makes 6 servings.

Ginger Pork

1 (2-1/2 pound) additive-free boneless pork roast, trimmed, cut
    into 1-inch pieces
2 tablespoons extra-virgin olive oil (more if needed)
1 cup chicken stock (see recipe)
1-1/2 tablespoons arrowroot starch / flour
3 tablespoons soy sauce substitute or Coconut Aminos (see recipe,
    note)
1 teaspoon fresh ginger, grated
1 (15-ounce) can pineapple chunks with juice
1 (16-ounce) package baby carrots
1 small can bamboo shoots, drained
White rice, cooked

Heat 1 tablespoon oil in large heavy skillet over medium-high heat.
Cook in several batches until browned on all sides, about 5 to 6
minutes total. Set aside to drain. In large slow cooker combine
chicken stock, soy sauce substitute or Coconut Aminos, ginger,
pineapple juice (not chunks), carrots and bamboo shoots. Place
pineapple chunks in refrigerator until ready for use. Add browned
pork to crock pot. Cover and cook on low 6 to 8 hours, stirring
several times. Cook rice according to directions on package. When
rice is ready, set aside in covered dish to keep warm. Turn crock pot
to high and stir in pineapple chunks. Cover and cook for an
additional 10 minutes. Turn crock pot off. In small bowl, whisk
arrowroot starch together with equal amount of cold water, and mix
in with contents of crock pot, stirring for 1 to 2 minutes, until juices
thicken Serve over hot, cooked rice. Makes 4 to 6 servings.

Coconut Aminos can be substituted for soy sauce in dressings,
marinades and other recipes. This product is not derived from the
nut of the coconut tree.

Pulled Pork

4 pounds additive-free pork roast (shoulder or butt only)
1 recipe Memphis Rub (or safe meat rub of choice)
2 large onions, sliced
1/4 cup apple cider vinegar
1-1/2 cups barbeque sauce, 1/2 cup reserved to serve with (see recipe)
Hamburger buns (optional, see recipe)
Hollowed-out baked potato skins (optional, see recipe)

Massage rub into meat. Wrap tightly in double layer of plastic wrap and refrigerate at least 3 hours, or for stronger flavor, refrigerate up to 3 days. Unwrap meat and place it in crock pot with onion slices placed around sides of roast. Add cider vinegar. Cover and cook on low 8 to 10 hours, until meat is fork-tender. Remove meat, strain and save onions. Discard liquid. With two forks, shred meat, discarding any remaining fat, bones or skin. Most of the fat will have melted away. Return shredded meat and the onions to crock pot. Stir in 1 cup barbeque sauce. Continue to cook on low another hour. Larger crock pots may cook faster, so cooking time may be reduced depending on tenderness. Serve with and hamburger buns and barbecue sauce, or for an interesting (and delicious) twist, spoon into hollowed out potato skins. Leftovers freeze well.

Roast Pork Shoulder

1 (6 pound) additive-free pork roast (shoulder)
8 cloves garlic, minced
1 tablespoon fresh rosemary, finely chopped
1 tablespoon sea salt
1 teaspoon freshly ground black pepper
Extra-virgin olive oil

Preheat oven to 350°F. In small bowl, mix garlic, rosemary, salt, pepper and enough olive oil to form a paste. With sharp knife, score the roast, cutting 1/4-inch deep in crosshatch lines. Poke deep cuts into the surface of the roast with the knife. Rub paste unto the cuts. Place pork in large roasting pan, and roast for 3 hours. Remove excess fat. Roast pork for 1-1/2 to 2 hours longer, until skin is crisp and dark brown. Remove from oven. Tent loosely with foil, and let rest 20 minutes. Remove pork skin and cut into small pieces. Slice meat. Serve hot or at room temperature with some of the pork skin. Makes 8 to 10 servings.

Roast Pork Tenderloin

1 additive-free bone-in pork tenderloin roast (2 ribs per person)
3 large onions
3 tablespoons fresh sage, chopped
3 tablespoons fresh thyme, chopped
Sea salt and freshly ground black pepper

Remove roast from refrigerator about 1 hour before cooking. Preheat oven to 450°F. Rub all sides of pork with sage and thyme. Sprinkle with salt and pepper. Cover ends of bones with aluminum foil to prevent from burning. Slice onions and place pork loin on top of them in ovenproof dish. Place in oven and reduce heat to 325°F. Cook 40 minutes per pound, basting frequently with pan juices. Remove from oven, loosely tent with foil and allow to rest 15 minutes before carving. Serving size depends on number of ribs per person.

Spice-Rubbed Pork Tenderloin

2 additive-free pork tenderloins (boneless, about 2 pounds total)
4 teaspoons pure cane dark brown sugar (see note)
1 tablespoon sea salt
1 teaspoon freshly ground black pepper
2-1/2 teaspoons sweet paprika
1-1/4 teaspoon smoked paprika
1/4 teaspoon ground cinnamon
1/8 teaspoon ground allspice
1/2 tablespoon extra-virgin olive oil

Position rack in center of oven and preheat to 450°F. Lightly oil a heavy rimmed baking sheet or ovenproof glass dish. Mix brown sugar, salt, pepper, sweet paprika, smoked paprika, cinnamon and allspice in a large bowl. Coat tenderloins evenly with rub mix. Roast the tenderloins for 10 minutes and then lower the oven temperature to 325°F. Continue cooking 25 to 30 minutes, or until meat thermometer inserted in the center of each tenderloin reads 140°F. Remove to a platter and let rest 5 minutes. Slice meat and serve hot. Makes 6 servings.

Dark brown sugar can be replaced with 1/2 cup white sugar and 2 tablespoons corn-free molasses or Yacon syrup for each 1/2 cup.

Wild Rice Stuffed Pork Chops

4 additive-free pork loin chops, 1-inch thick
1/3 cup corn-free apricot preserves
1 tablespoon dry white wine or apple juice
1/8 teaspoon ground cinnamon
1 tablespoon extra-virgin olive oil

Stuffing:
1/3 cup celery, finely chopped
1 green onion, finely chopped
1 teaspoon extra-virgin olive oil
1 cup cooked wild rice
1/4 teaspoon sea salt
1/8 teaspoon freshly ground black pepper

For stuffing, cook celery and onion in 1 teaspoon oil in heavy skillet over medium heat, stirring frequently, until celery is crisp-tender. Stir in remaining ingredients. Set aside in bowl. Preheat oven to 350°F. Heat 1 tablespoon oil in heavy skillet over medium heat. Cut deep pocket in each pork chop on side opposite the bone. Stuff about 1/3 cup stuffing mixture into each pocket. Mix apricot preserves, wine or apple juice, and cinnamon. Fasten edges with toothpicks. Season pork chops with salt and pepper. Place into hot skillet. Cook on each side until browned, about 3 minutes, then transfer to baking dish. Cover with aluminum foil. Bake in preheated oven until pork is no longer pink in center, about 40 minutes. When almost done, uncover and bake about 10 minutes longer. Makes 4 servings.

Rice

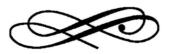

Fragrant Fried Rice

1-1/4 cups basmati rice
2-1/2 cups water (more if needed)
3 tablespoons extra-virgin olive oil
8 whole cloves
4 black cardamom pods, bruised
1 bay leaf
1 (3-inch) cinnamon stick
1 teaspoon black peppercorns
1 teaspoon cumin seeds
1 teaspoon coriander seeds
Sea salt to taste
1 small cauliflower, cut into tiny flowerets
1 onion, sliced into rings

Place rice in medium bowl, cover with water, and soak 30 minutes. Heat oil over medium-high in heavy skillet. Add cloves, cardamom pods, bay leaf, cinnamon, peppercorns, cumin seeds and coriander seeds and cook for 1 minute. Add onion and cook 5 minutes, stirring frequently, until tender. Drain rice and reserve liquid. Add rice to skillet and cook 2 to 3 minutes, until opaque and light golden. Stir in reserved water, salt and cauliflower. Bring to a boil, reduce heat and cover. Simmer 12 to 15 minutes, stirring occasionally, until all liquid is absorbed and rice and cauliflower are tender. Add water 1 tablespoon at a time if more is needed. Remove whole spices before serving. Makes 4 servings.

Red Beans and Rice

1 tablespoon extra-virgin olive oil (more if needed)
1 package Al Fresco Fresh Sweet Italian Style Chicken Sausages, cut
    in 1/2-inch slices
1 yellow onion, chopped
1 green Bell pepper
1 clove minced garlic
2 (16-ounce) cans dark red kidney beans, drained
1 (14-1/2-ounce) can stewed tomatoes, with juice (or see recipe)
1/2 teaspoon dried oregano
1/2 teaspoon dried parsley
1/2 teaspoon freshly ground black pepper
1 cup water
1/2 cup uncooked rice

It helps to partially freeze the sausages for about 30 minutes before
slicing. Heat oil in large skillet over medium heat. Cook sausage
slices until done and slightly browned, about 5 to 7 minutes. Stir in
onion, green pepper and garlic and sauté until onion is tender. Add
beans, stewed tomatoes and pepper. Cook until heated through,
stirring frequently, about 5 minutes. Add water and rice and stir.
Bring mixture to a boil, reduce heat and simmer covered 20
minutes. Makes 8 servings.

Saffron Rice Pudding

1-1/4 cups basmati rice
2-1/2 cups water
1/3 cup rice milk
1/8 teaspoon corn-free vanilla
Pinch of saffron threads
2 tablespoons grape seed oil
2 green cardamom pods, bruised
1 (1-inch) cinnamon stick
2 whole cloves
1/2 cup golden raisins
1/4 cup pure cane sugar

Place rice in a large saucepan with water. Bring to a boil, reduce heat and simmer 5 minutes. Remove from heat and drain. Measure 2 tablespoons rice milk into small bowl, add saffron and soak 5 minutes. Heat grape seed oil in heavy saucepan, add rice, cardamom pods, cinnamon and cloves and cook 2 to 3 minutes, or until rice becomes opaque. Stir in remaining rice milk, vanilla, saffron milk, raisins and sugar and bring to boil. Cover and simmer about 6 to 8 minutes, until rice is tender and liquid has been absorbed. Remove whole spices and serve hot. Makes 4 servings.

Sweet Saffron Rice

1-1/2 cups basmati rice
2-1/2 cups water
1 teaspoon saffron threads
3 tablespoons boiling water
3 tablespoons grape seed oil
6 whole cloves
6 green cardamom pods, bruised
1 (3-inch) stick cinnamon
1/2 cup raisins
3 tablespoons pure cane sugar
Pinch sea salt

Place rice in bowl with 2-1/2 cups water and soak 30 minutes. Put saffron in small bowl, add 3 tablespoons boiling water and soak. Heat oil in a heavy skillet over medium-high heat. Add cloves, cardamom pods and cinnamon and cook 1 minute. Drain rice and reserve water. Add rice to pan and cook until opaque and light golden, about 2 to 3 minutes. Stir in reserved water, saffron and the water it was soaking in, raisins, sugar and salt. Bring to a boil, reduce heat and cover. Simmer 12 to 15 minutes, stirring occasionally, until liquid is absorbed and rice is tender. Remove spices before serving. Serve hot. Makes 4 servings.

Wild Rice Pilaf

1 tablespoon extra-virgin olive oil
1/2 cup wild rice
1 cup long grain brown rice
1 medium onion, chopped
3/4 cup celery, diced into 1/2-inch pieces
2 cups crimini mushrooms, sliced
1 medium green apple, diced into 1/2-inch pieces
4 cloves garlic, minced
6 dried apricots, chopped
1/2 cup raisins
1/2 cup fresh parsley, chopped
2 tablespoon fresh sage, chopped
3 tablespoons fresh thyme, chopped
1/2 tablespoon fennel seeds
3/4 cup chicken stock (see recipe)
2 tablespoons extra-virgin olive oil (extra for drizzle)
Sea salt and black pepper to taste

Bring 3-1/2 cups lightly salted water to a boil. Rinse wild rice under
running water in strainer. When water is boiling, add wild rice and
brown rice, cover, turn heat to low, and cook about 45 minutes,
until tender.
There will most likely be excess water when rice is cooked properly.
Do not overcook. Put cooked rice in strainer and drain out excess
water. Set aside in a bowl large enough to mix everything together.
Preheat oven to 350°F. Heat 1 tablespoon olive oil in large stainless
steel skillet. Sauté onion over medium heat for 5 minutes. Add
mushrooms and celery and continue to sauté 2 to 3 minutes. Mix all
ingredients together except for onions and rice, and season with salt
and pepper. Fold into the rice mixture, followed next by the onion
mixture. Place blended mixture in an 8-inch square baking dish and
drizzle with reserved olive oil. Bake covered for about 1 hour. Mix
with a fork at 20 and 40 minutes to keep it fluffy. Goes great with
lamb or chicken. Makes 6 servings.

Salads

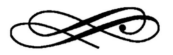

Avocado Salad ~ 143
Carrot Raisin Salad ~ 143
Caesar Salad ~ 144
Chicken Curry Salad ~ 145
Chicken Waldorf Salad ~ 145
Fresh Fruit Salad ~ 146
Mediterranean Chicken Salad ~ 147
Orange, Fennel and Avocado Salad ~ 148
Pineapple Salad with Ginger Syrup ~ 148
Potato Salad ~ 149
Quinoa Tabouleh ~ 150
Shredded Beet Salad with Raspberry Vinaigrette ~ 150
Summer Salad ~ 151

Avocado Salad

2 ripe avocados
2 tablespoons extra-virgin olive oil
2 tablespoons freshly squeezed lemon juice (about 1 lemon)
Sea salt and freshly ground black pepper to taste

Cut avocados in half. Twist to separate, and remove pits. Cut in half again lengthwise, then carefully peel skins off. Cut lengthwise one more time, so you wind up with thin wedges. Arrange on serving platter and drizzle with oil and lemon juice. Season with salt and pepper to taste. Makes 4 servings.

Carrot Raisin Salad

2 to 3 medium carrots (2 cups peeled and shredded)
1/2 cup raisins
1/2 cup fresh or canned pineapple chunks
1 tablespoon cilantro, chopped

Dressing:
2 tablespoons rice milk
1/4 teaspoon turmeric
1/2 tablespoon corn-free honey (see note)
1 teaspoon orange zest
1 tablespoon fresh lemon juice
1 tablespoon extra-virgin olive oil
Sea salt and freshly ground white pepper to taste

Blend all dressing ingredients together in blender adding the oil a little at a time at the end. Mix shredded carrots with raisins and pineapple, and toss with desired amount of dressing. Stir in chopped cilantro.

Always use caution when buying honey. Unless you buy certified 100% pure organic, it may contain unlabeled high fructose corn syrup. Honey can be replaced with agave nectar in many recipes.

Caesar Salad

1 package dark or 50/50 spring mix salad greens
Cooked additive-free chicken slices (optional)

Dressing:
2 tablespoons tahini
4 cloves garlic, minced
3 tablespoons lemon juice
2 tablespoons balsamic vinegar
2 tablespoons extra-virgin olive oil
Sea salt and freshly ground black pepper to taste

In blender, mix dressing ingredients together for 1 to 2 minutes, drizzling oil in last, a little at a time. Toss lettuce with desired amount of dressing. Add cooked chicken slices if desired. Dressing will keep up to 2 weeks in refrigerator. Makes about 1/2 cup of dressing.

Chicken Curry Salad

1-1/2 pounds additive-free chicken breasts, cooked and cut into
       1/2-inch cubes
1 tart apple, peeled, cored and diced
3 stalks celery, diced
1/2 cup golden raisins
1 tablespoon pure cane sugar
3/4 teaspoon curry powder
1/2 cup mayonnaise substitute (see recipe) or Soy Free Vegenaise
Salad greens (optional)
Sandwich bread (optional, see recipes)
Apple slices for garnish (optional)

In large bowl, whisk mayonnaise substitute or Soy Free Vegenaise,
curry powder, and sugar together until thoroughly blended. Add
diced apple, raisins and celery, and turn until coated. Add chicken
and mix well. Let marinate in tightly sealed container in refrigerator
several hours before serving. Serve on sandwich bread, or bed of
salad greens garnished with apple slices, if desired. Makes 4 to 6
servings. See caution, bottom of page 150.

Chicken Waldorf Salad

1-1/2 pounds additive-free chicken breast, cooked, cooled and cut
       into 1/2-inch cubes
3 tart apples, peeled, cored and diced
1 cup seedless grapes
3 stalks celery, diced
1/2 cup golden raisins
1 tablespoon pure cane sugar
1 tablespoon lemon juice
1/2 cup mayonnaise substitute (see recipe) or Soy Free Vegenaise

In large bowl, whisk mayonnaise substitute or Soy Free Vegenaise
with lemon juice and sugar together until thoroughly blended. Add
diced apples, grapes, celery and raisins and turn until coated. Add
chicken and mix well. Serve on bed of lettuce, if desired. Makes 4 to
6 servings. See caution, bottom of page 150.

Fresh Fruit Salad

1 cantaloupe, cut in half, and seeded
2 peaches, pitted, sliced, and then sliced in half
6 apricots, pitted and sliced
1 small bunch seedless grapes, stemmed
1/2 cup blueberries
2 tablespoons corn-free powdered sugar (see note)
1 orange, juiced
1 lemon, juiced
Lemon zest for garnish (optional)

Scoop out melon flesh into small balls and place in bowl. Remove
small slice on bottom of one half of melon shell so it sits flat on
plate, and discard other half. In large bowl, add melon balls,
peaches, apricots, grapes and blueberries. Sift sugar over the top
and sprinkle with orange and lemon juices. Stir well. Spoon mixture
into melon shell and garnish with lemon zest, if desired. Chill
before serving. Makes 4 servings.

Powdered sugar generally contains cornstarch. To make your own,
add 1 tablespoon potato starch to 1 cup of sugar and blend in a
coffee grinder until you get a fine texture.

Mediterranean Chicken Salad

1 pound boneless skinless additive-free chicken breast, sliced into
    thin strips
1 clove garlic, minced
1 large red onion, sliced
1/2 red Bell pepper, seeded and sliced into thin strips
1/2 yellow Bell pepper, seeded and sliced into thin strips
1 small zucchini, diced into 1/2-inch cubes
1 package (8-ounces) grape tomatoes
1 tablespoon extra-virgin olive oil (more for skillet)
2 tablespoon balsamic vinegar
1 tablespoon corn-free honey (see note)
1/2 teaspoon sea salt
Freshly ground black pepper to taste
12 black brined olives, pitted and cut into quarters (see note)
8 leaves fresh basil
8 romaine lettuce leaves

Preheat oven to 350°F. Combine minced garlic and chicken breast
strips in bowl, and refrigerate. Place large non-stick skillet in oven.
While skillet is heating, heat oil in second skillet over medium-high
heat on stove. Add onions, sauté until they begin to brown. Add
pepper strips and cook 5 to 7 minutes, mixing a few times. Remove
before peppers get too soft. Place zucchini and grape tomatoes on
skillet in oven, and place back in oven. Bake 5 to 7 minutes, mixing
twice to make sure they are well seared. Remove before the
tomatoes get soft and place in a large bowl to cool in refrigerator.
Shut oven off. Coat stove-top skillet with oil and add garlic and
chicken strips. Cook about 10 minutes, mixing several times, until
chicken is cooked through. Remove and add to roasted vegetable
mixture, mixing well to coat. Add 1 tablespoon olive oil, balsamic
vinegar, honey, salt, pepper, olives and basil. Mix to coat salad well
and marinate in refrigerator at least 2 hours. When ready to serve,
cut romaine lettuce into strips and fold into salad. Makes 4 servings.

Make sure the olives are brined with white wine vinegar, not
distilled white vinegar, which may contain corn or gluten. See honey
caution on bottom of page 144.

Orange, Fennel and Avocado Salad

2 tablespoons white wine vinegar
1/2 teaspoon sea salt
1/4 teaspoon freshly ground black pepper
1/4 cup extra-virgin olive oil
1 Naval orange or Blood orange
1 fennel bulb, stalks cut off and discarded
1 avocado, pit and peel removed, and cut into slices
Bed of lettuce (optional)

In medium bowl, whisk vinegar, salt, pepper and olive oil together.
Halve the orange lengthwise, then cut crosswise into thin slices.
Halve the fennel lengthwise, remove core, then cut crosswise into
thin slices. Carefully toss orange, fennel and avocado slices with
dressing. Serve on a bed of lettuce, if desired. Makes 2 to 4 servings.

Pineapple Salad with Ginger Syrup

1 cup water
1/4 cup corn-free honey (see note)
1/4 cup fresh ginger, peeled and thinly sliced
1 medium pineapple cut into 1-inch chunks
4 firm bananas, sliced

Combine water, honey and ginger in small saucepan over high heat.
Cook about 15 minutes, until mixture reduces and becomes syrupy.
Strain and refrigerate until completely cool, about 30 to 45 minutes.
Mixture will thicken slightly as it chills. Cut pineapple and banana
and mix together with chilled syrup. Makes 4 servings.

Always use caution when buying honey. Unless you buy certified
100% pure organic, it may contain unlabeled high fructose corn
syrup. Honey can be replaced with agave nectar in many recipes.

Potato Salad

2 pounds russet potatoes
2 stalks celery, finely chopped
1/4 cup onion, finely chopped
1 cup mayonnaise substitute (see recipe) or Soy Free Vegenaise
2 tablespoons corn-free sweet pickle relish (or see recipe)
4 teaspoons pure cane sugar
2 teaspoons prepared yellow mustard
1 teaspoon white wine vinegar
1/2 teaspoon freshly ground black pepper
1 teaspoon celery seed
Sea salt to taste
Paprika for garnish (optional)

Bring large saucepan of water to boil. Add salt and potatoes, reduce heat to medium-low and cook until tender but firm, about 15 minutes. Drain water, allow potatoes to cool and chop into pieces (about 1-inch square). Place potatoes, celery and onion in a large bowl and toss carefully to combine. In small bowl, combine mayonnaise substitute or Soy Free Vegenaise, relish, sugar, mustard, vinegar, pepper, celery seed and salt. Add dressing mixture to bowl with potatoes and mix carefully until coated with dressing. Refrigerate at least 2 hours (or overnight) before serving. Sprinkle with paprika if desired. Makes 8 servings.

Caution: Although the pea protein in Soy Free Vegenaise is not hydrolyzed, it may still contain enough naturally occurring free glutamate to serve as an MSG-trigger in highly sensitive people.

Quinoa Tabouleh

1 cup uncooked quinoa
2 cups water
1 cup Italian parsley, finely chopped
1/2 cup fresh mint leaves, finely chopped
1 pint grape or cherry tomatoes, cut in halves or quarters
1/2 cup chopped red onion
2 cloves garlic, minced
1 lemon, juiced
1-1/2 tablespoons extra-virgin olive oil
Sea salt to taste

Bring water to a boil in medium saucepan. Add quinoa, cover, and return to a boil. Reduce heat and simmer 15 minutes. Remove from heat and let stand 10 minutes. Remove lid and fluff with fork. Allow to cool completely in refrigerator before mixing with rest of ingredients. Mix quinoa with remaining ingredients in a large bowl. Let flavors marinate in refrigerate at least 1 hour before serving. Makes 6 to 8 servings.

Shredded Beet Salad with Raspberry Vinaigrette

5 orange beets, raw
1/2 cup fresh raspberries, rinsed, plus 1/4 cup reserved
2 tablespoon balsamic vinegar
4 tablespoons extra-virgin olive oil
2 tablespoons sunflower seeds, shelled
1 teaspoon pure cane sugar (more or less to taste)

Puree 1/2 cup of fresh raspberries in a blender or food processor. Add vinegar and oil. Blend well. Add sugar, blending a little at a time, to taste. Set aside in refrigerator. Shred beets in food processor and transfer to bowl. Coat beet mixture with vinaigrette mixture. Sprinkle with sunflower seeds and remaining 1/4 cup raspberries. Makes 4 to 6 servings.

Summer Salad

1 can (14-1/2-ounces) French style green beans, drained
1 can (14-1/2-ounces) baby peas, drained
1 can (14-1/2-ounces) sliced carrots, drained
1 yellow Bell pepper, seeded and diced
1 cup celery, diced thin
1 medium yellow onion, peeled and diced
1 jar (8 ounces or so) pimentos, drained

Marinade:
1-1/2 cups apple cider vinegar
2 tablespoons water
1 cup pure cane sugar
1 cup canola oil

Place all vegetables, fresh and canned, in a large mixing bowl, and toss carefully but well to combine. Set aside. In medium saucepan, combine all marinade ingredients, and bring to a boil over medium-high heat, mixing frequently until sugar dissolves, about 3 to 5 minutes. Remove from heat and set aside. Prepare container(s) for storing salad. I like to use a recycled 1-quart (64 ounce) pickle jar. Fill container(s) with vegetable mixture, taking care not to pack them down. Once container(s) are filled, pour marinade while still reasonably hot over vegetable mixture. Seal container(s) tightly and store in refrigerator at least 24 hours before use to let flavors marinate. Lasts several months in the refrigerator.

Soups, Stews and Stocks

Baby Carrot and Fennel Soup

1 tablespoon extra-virgin olive oil
1 small bunch scallions, chopped
1 bulb fennel, chopped
1 stalk celery, chopped
1 pound baby carrots, grated
1/2 teaspoon ground cumin
2 medium potatoes, diced small
5 cups chicken or vegetable stock (see recipe)
Sea salt and freshly ground black pepper
Fresh parsley, chopped for garnish (optional)

Heat oil over medium-high heat in medium saucepan. Add
scallions, fennel, celery, carrots and cumin. Stir well and reduce heat
to low. Cover and cook until soft, about 5 minutes. Add potatoes
and stock. Increase heat to medium, bring to a boil, then lower heat,
re-cover the pan, and simmer for 10 more minutes, until the
potatoes are soft. Remove from heat and let cool slightly. Puree
until smooth in blender or food processor. Season with salt and
pepper to taste. Serve hot, garnished with chopped parsley if
desired. Makes 4 servings.

Beef Stock

5 pounds meaty additive-free beef stock bones (with lots of
    marrow)
1 pound of additive-free beef stew meat or beef scraps, cut into
chunks
Extra-virgin olive oil
2 medium onions, peeled and quartered
4 carrots, chopped into 1 inch chunks
1 large, very ripe meaty tomato
2 stalks celery, including tops, cut into 1-inch chunks
3 cloves of garlic
1/3 cup fresh parsley, chopped
2 bay leaves
10 peppercorns

Preheat oven to 400°F. Rub oil over meat pieces, carrots, and
onions. Place in large, shallow roasting pan. Roast, uncovered,
about 30 minutes or until the bones are well browned, turning
occasionally. When bones are nicely browned, remove and place in
large stock pot. Place roasting pan over two burners on stove top
on low heat, pour 1 cup hot water over pan and scrape up browned
bits. Pour browned bits and water into large saucepan. Add celery,
garlic, parsley, bay leaves, and peppercorns. Fill with cold water to 1
to 2 inches over the top of bones. Bring to a boil, then reduce heat
to low and simmer, partially covered, 6 hours. Occasionally strain
away any fat and scum that rises to surface. Let set until cool
enough to handle, but still rather warm. Strain stock. Discard meat,
vegetables, and seasonings. Chill, and remove any fat that rises to
the top and solidifies. Makes roughly 4 quarts.

Carrot Ginger Bisque

2 tablespoons extra-virgin olive oil
1 large onion
1/8 cup garlic, minced
3 pounds carrots, diced, with skin left on
1-1/2 pounds butternut squash, cubed
1-1/2 quarts chicken stock (see recipe)
1/2 quart pulpy orange juice
1 bay leaf
1/4 teaspoons freshly ground white pepper
1/4 tablespoon sea salt
1/4 cup fresh ginger, grated
1/8 teaspoon nutmeg (more for garnish)
1/8 teaspoon thyme, ground

Heat oil in heavy saucepan. Add onions and brown slightly. Add garlic and sauté until aromatic, 1 to 2 minutes. Add carrots, squash, stock, orange juice and bay leaf. Cook until carrots and squash are tender enough to puree. Puree soup and add rest of ingredients. Serve hot with pinch of nutmeg on top, if desired. Makes 6 to 8 servings.

Chicken Stew

2 pounds additive-free chicken breast, skinned, cut into chunks
2 tablespoons extra-virgin olive oil
1 large onion, peeled and chopped
1 cup mushrooms, chopped
2 cloves garlic, minced
1 tablespoon fresh thyme
1/2 teaspoon freshly ground black pepper
1/4 teaspoon sea salt
2 bay leaves
4 cups chicken stock (see recipe)
1/2 cup white wine
4 medium carrots, cut into 1-inch chunks
4 parsnips, peeled and cut into 1-inch chunks
1/2 cup white bean flour
1/2 cup cold water
White rice or Spinach and Bean Dumplings (optional, see recipe)

Heat half the oil in medium saucepan over medium heat. Cook chicken in batches until lightly browned, about 8 to 10 minutes, turning often. Add rest of oil if needed. Remove chicken and set aside. Add onion, mushrooms, garlic, thyme, salt, pepper and bay leaves. Cook 4 to 5 minutes, until vegetables begin to brown. Stir in chicken stock and white wine. Add carrots and parsnips. Return chicken to saucepan. Bring to a boil, cover and reduce heat. Simmer 30 to 35 minutes, or until chicken and vegetables are tender. Using a slotted spoon, transfer chicken and vegetables to serving dish and keep warm. Remove excess fat and bay leaves from broth mixture. Whisk white bean flour in small bowl with 1/2 cup cold water. Mix into stew, stirring constantly. Continue to whisk until stew thickens, another 3 to 5 minutes. If you desire a thicker stew, whisk equal amounts of white bean four with water, and add to stew one or two tablespoons at a time until desired consistency is reached. Spoon thickened broth over chicken and vegetables. May be served alone as a stew, or with white rice and Spinach and Bean Dumplings, if desired. Makes 4 servings.

Chicken Stock

1 tablespoon extra-virgin olive oil
2 medium carrots, chopped
1 stalk celery, including leaves, chopped
1 large onion, peeled and chopped
6 cups water
1 small (3 pound) additive-free chicken, skinned and quartered,
    excess fat removed, or meaty carcass and meat from 1 larger,
    picked over chicken
1 cup mushrooms, chopped
1/4 cup fresh parsley, chopped
2 bay leaves
10 black peppercorns
2 whole cloves
1/4 teaspoon freshly ground white pepper

Heat oil in large saucepan over medium heat. Add carrot, celery and onion. Cook, stirring often, until onion is golden, about 10 minutes. Add water, chicken, mushrooms, parsley, bay leaf, peppercorns and cloves. Bring to a boil over high heat, then reduce and simmer, partially covered, 2 hours. Add white pepper, remove from heat and let cool slightly. When cool enough to handle, but still relatively warm, strain and discard solids. When fully cooled off, refrigerate, and remove any fat that has risen to top and solidified. Makes roughly 4 to 5 cups.

Chilled Tomato and Sweet Pepper Soup

2 red Bell peppers, halved and seeded
3 tablespoons extra-virgin olive oil
1 onion, finely chopped
2 garlic cloves, crushed
2 large ripe tomatoes
2/3 cup red wine
2-1/2 cups chicken stock (see recipe)
Sea salt and freshly ground black pepper

Place Bell peppers skin side up on broiler rack and broil on low
heat until skins are charred. Transfer to bowl and cover tightly.
Heat oil over medium in large saucepan. Add onion and garlic and
cook until tender, stirring frequently, about 5 minutes. Uncover
bowl containing peppers. Remove skins and chop into large chunks.
Cut tomatoes into large chunks. Add peppers and tomatoes to pan.
Cover, reduce heat to medium low and simmer 10 minutes. Add
wine and cook another 5 minutes. Add stock, season with salt and
pepper, and simmer another 20 minutes. Allow to cool, and process
in blender or food processor until smooth. Chill in refrigerator at
least 3 hours before serving. Makes 4 servings.

Cream of Chicken Soup

2 cups additive-free chicken, cooked and diced
2 tablespoons extra-virgin olive oil
1 sprig fresh basil
1 medium onion, chopped
1 sprig fresh oregano
1 clove garlic, minced
1 bay leaf
2 stalks celery, chopped
5 cups chicken stock (see recipe)
1 cup rice milk, room temperature
1 cup carrots, diced
1 cup white bean flour
Sea salt and freshly ground black pepper

Heat oil in a large saucepan over medium heat. Add onion, garlic, celery and carrots and cook, covered, stirring occasionally until tender, about 12 minutes. Drain any extra oil. In same pan, combine stock, oregano, basil and bay leaf. Bring to a boil, reduce heat to medium-low, cover and simmer 15 minutes. Stir in chicken and bring to a boil. Whisk bean flour in a small bowl with rice milk. Mix into soup, stirring constantly. Continue to whisk until stew thickens, another 3 to 5 minutes. Remove from heat. Add salt and pepper to taste. Serve hot. Makes 6 servings.

Cream of Mushroom Soup

2 tablespoons extra-virgin olive oil
4 cups button mushrooms, sliced
3 cups beef stock (see recipe)
3 cups rice milk, 1 cup reserved
2 medium shallots, chopped
3 tablespoons cream sherry
1 cup white bean flour
Sea salt and freshly ground black pepper

Heat oil in a large skillet over medium heat. Add shallots and sliced mushrooms. Sauté about 5 to 10 minutes, until shallots are tender and mushrooms begin to brown. Add sherry and continue to cook until liquid evaporates. In large saucepan, combine beef stock, 2 cups rice milk, salt and pepper and bring to boil. Reduce heat to medium-low. Add shallot and mushroom mixture. Stir well, and cook 5 more minutes. Whisk bean flour in a small bowl with 1 cup reserved rice milk. Mix into soup, stirring constantly. Continue to whisk until stew thickens, another 3 to 5 minutes. Add salt and pepper to taste. Serve hot. Makes 4 servings.

Split Pea Soup with Ham

1-1/2 cups dried green split peas, rinsed and drained
6 cups water or vegetable stock, more if needed (see recipe)
2 tablespoons extra-virgin olive oil
2 medium leeks, thinly sliced
2 medium potatoes, peeled and thinly sliced
2 medium carrots, thinly sliced
2 stalks celery, thinly sliced
1 tablespoon fresh thyme
1 bay leaf
1 cup young green peas, fresh or frozen
1/4 teaspoon sea salt
1/4 teaspoon freshly ground white pepper
1 additive-free ham bone with meat attached

Place peas in large saucepan with ham bone and water or stock. If liquid doesn't cover one, add just enough to cover it. Bring to boil, then reduce heat to low and simmer, covered, 1 hour. Heat oil in large skillet over medium heat. Add leeks and sauté until soft, stirring occasionally, about 5 minutes. Add to saucepan, along with potatoes, carrots, celery, thyme and bay leaf. Bring to a boil, then reduce and simmer, covered, about 30 minutes. Remove from heat and let set until cool enough to handle. Remove bay leaf and discard. Remove bone, take off the meat and chop it finely. Set meat aside and discard ham bone. Transfer soup mixture to blender or food processor, and process to coarse texture. Return to saucepan. Add meat, green peas, salt and pepper. Bring to a boil over medium heat, reduce heat to low and simmer, covered, until peas are tender, about 5 minutes. Serve hot. Makes 8 servings.

Stewed Tomatoes

2 large tomatoes, cut into 1-inch chunks
1/2 cup water
1/4 cup chopped onion
2 tablespoons Coconut Aminos (see note)
2 teaspoons pure cane sugar
1 teaspoon extra-virgin olive oil
1/2 teaspoon sea salt (more to taste)
1/4 teaspoon dried basil
1/4 teaspoon dried parsley

In medium saucepan over medium-high heat, add olive oil, chopped tomatoes, onion and water. Stir until mixture begins to simmer, stirring frequently. Add rest of ingredients, reduce heat to a gentle simmer, and cook until tomatoes are tender and have lost their shape, about 10 to 15 minutes, stirring occasionally. Season with more salt to taste. Makes about 3 cups of stewed tomatoes. Freeze well.

Coconut Aminos can be substituted for soy sauce in dressings, marinades and other recipes. This product is not derived from the nut of the coconut tree.

Note: Both of these recipes are good to make in larger batches and freeze for later use. Since most of the recipes in this book that call for stewed tomatoes or tomato sauce do so in 1 cup measurements, I would suggest freezing them in 1 cup batches.

Tomato Sauce

Using the same ingredients from the Stewed Tomatoes recipe, above, prepare everything the same, except remove and discard the seeds from the tomatoes before chopping them. Once everything has been added to the saucepan, simmer twice as long, uncovered, about 30 minutes, stirring occasionally. After you season it to taste, let the tomatoes cool for about 15 to 20 minutes. Transfer to a blender, and process until smooth. Makes about 3 cups of tomato sauce for use in recipes. Freezes well. See note, above.

Turkey Carcass Stock

Leftover carcass of 1 (12 to 14 pound) additive-free turkey
1 onion, quartered
1/4 teaspoon peppercorns
1 leaf fresh thyme
1 bay leaf

Break leftover turkey carcass into 4 pieces. Place carcass, along with any other leftover bones in bottom of large stockpot. Add onion, peppercorns, thyme and bay leaf. Cover with approximately 1 gallon cold water. Bring to boil, reduce heat to medium-low and simmer, skimming the surface occasionally, until stock is concentrated in flavor, about 3 hours. Strain stock into second saucepan and simmer until reduced by almost half, 1 to 2 hours longer. Use in recipes as needed, or let cool and freeze in serving size sealable plastic bags for later use. Makes roughly 2 quarts.

Turkey Stock

Backbone, neck, wings from 18 pound additive-free turkey, or 6
        pounds additive-free turkey wings
6 quarts water
4 garlic cloves
2 stalks celery
1 carrot, peeled and thickly sliced
1 onion, quartered
1/4 teaspoon peppercorns
2 sprigs parsley
1 thyme
1 bay leaf

Combine all ingredients in large saucepan and bring to a boil. Reduce heat to medium-low and simmer, skimming as necessary, until stock is flavorful and reduced to 12 cups, about 3 hours. Strain stock and skim off fat. Can be made several days ahead. Also freezes well for future use. For even greater convenience, freeze in serving sized sealable bags. Makes 12 cups.

Vegetable Stock

1 tablespoon extra-virgin olive oil
2 medium carrots, thinly sliced
2 stalks celery, including leaves, thinly sliced
1 cup turnip or butternut squash, cubed
1 large onion, peeled and chopped
6 cups water
1 cup mushrooms, chopped
1/4 cup fresh parsley, chopped
1 bay leaf
10 black peppercorns
2 whole cloves
1/4 teaspoon freshly ground white pepper

Heat oil in large saucepan over medium heat. Add carrot, celery and onion. Cook, stirring often, until onion is golden, about 10 minutes. Add water, turnip or squash, mushrooms, parsley, bay leaf, peppercorns and cloves. Bring to a boil over high heat, then reduce and simmer, partially covered, for 2 hours. Add white pepper, remove from heat and let cool slightly. When cool enough to handle, but still relatively warm, strain and discard solids. When fully cooled off, refrigerate, and remove any fat that has risen to top and solidified. Use in recipes as needed, or let cool and freeze in serving size sealable plastic bags for later use. Makes roughly 4 to 5 cups.

Turkey and Stuffing

Bread Stuffing

1-1/2 loaves bread (see recipes)
4 tablespoons extra-virgin olive oil, plus more to grease pan
2 onions, diced
2 stalks celery, diced
1/2 cup diced carrot
2 shallots, minced
2 teaspoons rubbed sage
2 teaspoons dried thyme
2 teaspoons sea salt
1 teaspoon freshly ground pepper
1/2 cup white wine
1-1/2 cups chicken stock, more or less as needed (see recipe)

Preheat the oven to 300°F. Lightly grease baking sheet with oil. Cut bread into 1/2-inch cubes and place on sheet in single layer. Toast in oven until lightly browned, about 45 minutes, tossing every 15 minutes to ensure even toasting. When dried completely, remove from oven and cool. Increase oven temperature to 325°F. Heat oil over medium heat in large skillet. Add onions, celery, carrot and shallots and sauté until tender, about 6 to 8 minutes. Add sage, thyme, salt and pepper and cook an additional 2 minutes, stirring frequently. Add wine and continue to cook until wine is reduced by half. In large bowl, add toasted bread cubes and vegetable mixture, and toss to combine. Add chicken stock a little at a time, and stir until the bread cubes are evenly moistened. You may need more or less stock, depending on the type of bread used. You don't want it to be soupy. Once you get it to the right consistency, either transfer to baking dish and bake 20 to 25 minutes, or use as an actual stuffing for your turkey. 8 to 10 servings, or about enough for a 10 to 12 pound turkey. You may need to adjust amounts depending on size of turkey.

NOTE: Always stuff turkey just before roasting, never ahead of time, to avoid growth of harmful bacteria. Make sure the stuffing is hot, and pack it loosely in the body cavity.

Spinach, Fennel and Sausage Stuffing

1 loaf bread, cut into 1-inch cubes (see recipes)
2 tablespoons extra-virgin olive oil
1 package Al Fresco Fresh Sweet Italian Style Chicken Sausages
1 yellow onion, chopped
1 medium fennel bulb, cored and chopped
2 cups chicken stock, more or less as needed (see recipe)
2 pounds frozen spinach, thawed, drained and chopped
2 teaspoons sea salt
1-1/2 teaspoons freshly ground black pepper
1-1/2 teaspoons fennel seeds

Preheat to 350°F. Spread bread cubes out on rimmed baking sheet. Toast in oven 10 to 15 minutes, tossing once, until golden brown. Remove and set aside to cool. Remove casings from sausages and reserve meat. Heat 1 tablespoon oil over medium-high heat in large skillet. Add sausage and cook, breaking up into pieces and stirring frequently until browned, 8 to10 minutes. Remove and set aside to drain on paper towels. Add remaining oil to skillet and heat over medium-high heat. Add onion and fennel and cook, stirring occasionally, until soft, 10 to12 minutes. Grease shallow, oven-proof baking dish. Place sausage, onion and fennel mixture, spinach, salt, pepper, and fennel seeds in large bowl and mix well. Add chicken and the bread, and stir. Add 3/4 of the stock, and toss to coat evenly. Add rest of stock a little at a time, taking care not to let the mixture, and especially the bread, become soupy. Toss mixture until evenly distributed and bread has absorbed all the liquid. Either transfer to prepared baking dish and bake until stuffing is hot and the top is golden brown, about 40 minutes, or use as an actual stuffing for your turkey. Makes 8 to 10 servings, or about enough for a 10 to 12 pound turkey. You may need to adjust amounts depending on size of turkey.

NOTE: Always stuff turkey just before roasting, never ahead of time, to avoid growth of harmful bacteria. Make sure the stuffing is hot, and pack it loosely in the body cavity.

Traditional Roast Turkey

1 (18 pound) additive-free turkey
1/4 cup extra-virgin olive oil
Sea salt and freshly ground black pepper to taste
6 cups turkey stock (see recipe)
8 cups prepared stuffing (optional)

If the turkey has been refrigerated, you will need to bring it to room temperature in its plastic wrapping before preparing and cooking it. Keep it on a rimmed pan to collect any leaks. If the turkey is frozen, you will need to defrost it in the refrigerator for several days before you can cook it. It takes about 5 hours for every pound to defrost, so an 18 pound turkey would take about 90 hours in the refrigerator, or just under 4 days.

When handling raw turkey, use a separate cutting board and utensils to avoid contaminating other foods. Wash your hands with soap before touching anything else in the kitchen, and use paper towels to clean up.

Preheat oven to 325°F. Place rack in lowest position of oven. Remove turkey neck and giblets, and reserve neck, heart and gizzards for gravy, if desired. Rinse turkey both inside and out, and pat dry with paper towels. Place turkey breast side up on rack in roasting pan. If using stuffing, loosely fill body cavity with stuffing. Using a pastry brush, coat skin with oil, and season with salt and pepper. Tent loosely with aluminum foil. Place turkey in oven, and pour 2 cups turkey stock into bottom of roasting pan. Baste every 30 minutes with juices from bottom of the pan. Whenever the drippings evaporate, add more stock to moisten them, about 1 to 2 cups at a time. Remove aluminum foil after 2-1/2 hours. Roast until meat thermometer inserted in meaty part of thigh reads 180°F, about 4 hours. Transfer turkey to large serving platter, and let stand 20 to 30 minutes before carving. Makes 16 to 20 servings.

NOTE: Always stuff turkey just before roasting, never ahead of time, to avoid growth of harmful bacteria. Make sure the stuffing is hot, and pack it loosely in the body cavity.

Turkey Breakfast Sausage

3 tablespoons extra-virgin olive oil
1 medium onion, finely chopped
1 clove garlic, minced
2 pounds freshly ground additive-free turkey
1 tablespoon fennel seed
2 teaspoons ground sage
1 teaspoon sea salt
1/2 teaspoon freshly ground black pepper
1/8 teaspoon red pepper flakes

Heat 1 tablespoon oil over medium-high heat in large skillet. Add
onion and garlic, sauté onion until tender, about 5 minutes. Remove
from heat. Mix turkey, fennel seed, sage, salt, pepper and red
pepper flakes in medium bowl. Add onion and garlic mixture. Using
your hands, knead ingredients together well. Measure 1/4 cup of
turkey mixture and form into a round patty about 1/2-inch thick.
Form rest of turkey mixture into patties. Heat 1 tablespoon oil over
medium-high heat in large skillet. Working in batches, add patties
and cook 5 to 6 minutes on each side. Add more oil as needed.
Makes approximately 12 to 15 patties.

These freeze well. You might want to consider making a double
batch, and saving some for later use. To reheat, microwave 1
minute per patty. Can also be stuffed into sausage casings to create
a more traditional sausage shape, if desired.

Turkey Gravy

6 cups turkey stock (see recipe)
2 large carrots, chopped in large pieces
2 medium onions, cut into large pieces
2 celery sticks, cut into large pieces
Neck and gizzards from additive-free turkey (optional)
1 tablespoon fresh rosemary, chopped
2 tablespoons fresh thyme, chopped
1/4 cup dried porcini mushrooms (optional)
Sea salt and freshly ground black pepper
1 tablespoon potato starch for each cup of stock (about 3/8 cup)

In a large saucepan over medium heat, add stock, carrots, onions, celery, neck and gizzards if using, rosemary, thyme and mushrooms, if using, and simmer uncovered for about 1 hour. Strain and discard solids. If you are using gizzards and prefer to keep them, discard neck, and dice rest of gizzards into tiny pieces and return to saucepan. Reduce heat to medium-low, add rosemary and simmer another 20 minutes, stirring occasionally. Season to taste with chopped thyme, salt, and pepper. Cool and refrigerate until you remove turkey from oven. While turkey is resting, heat gravy over medium-high heat until it begins to a simmer, and remove from heat. In a small bowl, mix equal parts potato starch and cold water, and whisk well. Slowly pour into gravy a little at a time while stirring constantly. Do this just before serving, and do not boil the gravy once the potato starch has been added. Add more or less as desired, for a thinner or thicker gravy. You would want to double this recipe for an 18 pound turkey. Makes approximately 8 servings.

Turkey Jambalaya

8-ounces boneless, skinless additive-free turkey breast, cut into 1-
    inch pieces
2 limes, juiced
1 tablespoon fresh oregano, chopped, plus extra for garnish
1/4 teaspoon freshly ground white pepper
1 tablespoon plus 1 teaspoon extra-virgin olive oil
1 small onion, coarsely chopped
1 clove garlic, minced
1-1/2 cups mushrooms, thickly sliced
1 large tomato, coarsely chopped
1 cup long grain rice
1/2 cup okra, thickly sliced
1-3/4 cups hot chicken stock (see recipe)
1/2 cup green Bell pepper, thinly sliced
1/2 cup red Bell pepper, thinly sliced
1 tablespoon capers

Place cubed turkey in shallow glass dish. Pour lime juice on top,
then coat with 1 tablespoon oregano and white pepper. Toss to
coat, then cover and place in refrigerator. Heat rest of oil in a large
skillet over medium-high heat. Add onion and garlic, and sauté until
softened, about 5 minutes. Add turkey and cook, stirring constantly
until lightly browned, about 4 to 6 minutes. Add mushrooms,
tomato, rice and okra. Pour in hot chicken stock. Cover and cook
over medium-low heat until rice is almost tender, about 25 minutes.
Stir in Bell peppers, cover and cook until rice is tender, about 10
more minutes. Stir in capers, and sprinkle the remaining oregano on
top. Serve immediately. Makes 4 servings.

Wild Rice and Fruit Stuffing

1/2 cup wild rice
1 cup long grain brown rice
3-1/2 cups water
1 tablespoon extra-virgin olive oil
1 medium onion, chopped
3 stalks celery, chopped
2 cups fresh crimini mushrooms, sliced
1 tart apple, peeled and diced
4 cloves garlic, minced
1/4 cup plump dried apricots, chopped
1/2 cup golden raisins
1/2 cup dried cranberries
1/2 cup chopped fresh parsley
2 tablespoons chopped fresh sage
3 tablespoons chopped fresh thyme
1/2 cup plus 1 tablespoon turkey or chicken stock (see recipe)
Sea salt and freshly ground black pepper to taste

Bring 3-1/2 cups of lightly salted water to a boil. Add wild and
brown rice, cover, reduce heat to low and cook about 45 minutes,
until tender. Put cooked rice in strainer and drain out excess water.
Set aside in large bowl. Heat oil over medium-high heat in large
skillet. Add onion and sauté until tender and starts to turn golden,
about 5 minutes. Add mushrooms and celery, and sauté 2 to 3
minutes. Add to bowl with rest of ingredients, and mix well. Season
with salt and pepper. At this point, you can either cover and
refrigerate in microwave-safe dish until ready for use as a side
stuffing, or use as an actual stuffing for your turkey. Makes 8 to 10
servings, or about enough for a 10 to 12 pound turkey. You may
need to adjust amounts depending on size of turkey.

NOTE: Always stuff turkey just before roasting, never ahead of
time, to avoid growth of harmful bacteria. Make sure the stuffing is
hot, and pack it loosely in the body cavity.

Vegetables

Baked Eggplant

4 eggplants, cut lengthwise in half
1 tablespoon sea salt
4 cloves garlic, minced
4 onions, thinly sliced
1 cup extra-virgin olive oil
2 large ripe tomatoes, finely chopped
1 tablespoon fresh parsley, finely chopped (optional)

Make several long cuts in the sliced side of eggplants. Place in strainer, sprinkle with salt, and let drain for 1 hour. Preheat oven to 350°F. Heat 2 tablespoons oil in large skillet over medium heat and cook garlic and onions until lightly browned, about 8 to 10 minutes. Season with salt. Add tomatoes and simmer 15 minutes. Heat remaining oil in large skillet over medium high heat until very hot. Fry eggplants until flesh has softened, 10 to 15 minutes. Place eggplants in baking dish and fill with onion tomato mixture. Bake until tender, about 25 to 30 minutes. Sprinkle with parsley and serve hot. Makes 4 servings.

Broccoli Salad

1 head broccoli, trimmed into bite-sized flowerets
1/2 pound additive-free bacon, drained and crumbled
1/2 cup red onion, chopped
1/2 cup golden raisins
1 cup mayonnaise substitute (see recipe) or Soy Free Vegenaise
2 tablespoons white wine vinegar
1/4 cup pure cane sugar
1/4 cup shelled sunflower seeds
Sea salt and freshly ground black pepper

Place broccoli flowerets in large bowl. Add crumbled bacon, onion, raisins and sunflower seeds. In small bowl, whisk remaining ingredients together. Add to broccoli mixture and toss gently. Flavor comes out more if you refrigerate several hours, or even overnight. Toss well before serving. Makes 6 to 8 servings.

Caution: Although the pea protein in Soy Free Vegenaise is not hydrolyzed, it may still contain enough naturally occurring free glutamate to serve as an MSG-trigger in highly sensitive people.

Caramelized Onions

4 tablespoons extra-virgin olive oil (more if needed)
6 medium sweet onions, cut into rings
1 tablespoon pure cane sugar
Pinch of sea salt
Splash of water, stock or red wine as needed (for stock see recipes)

Coat bottom of heavy skillet with oil and heat over medium-high heat until shimmering. Add onions and stir well, coating onions with oil. Add salt and sugar, and stir well. Reduce heat to medium-low. Cook, stirring every few minutes, for 30 to 40 minutes, until onions are a deep caramel color. If they start to stick to the bottom of the pan too much, add a small amount of water, stock or wine, and stir vigorously; this is called "deglazing." The liquid will evaporate almost immediately while loosening the onion slices. Continue this process of cooking and deglazing until onions have reached the color, flavor, and texture you desire. May be made in advance if kept in an airtight container in the refrigerator. They also freeze well. An easy way to do it is freeze them in ice cube trays, then transfer to a sealable plastic bag until ready to use. This is one of those recipes you might want to double just so you can have some on hand later. Makes 2-1/2 to 3 cups.

Serving suggestions: Baked potatoes, burgers, chicken cutlets, cooked pasta, couscous, mashed potatoes, pan sauces, pizza, pork chops, risotto, sausages, sautéed vegetables, spinach salad, steaks, stews and soups.

Caramelized Onion-Stuffed Baked Potatoes

1/2 recipe caramelized onions (see recipe)
3 medium baking potatoes
1 tablespoon extra-virgin olive oil
1/2 teaspoon sea salt
1/4 teaspoon freshly ground black pepper
1/4 teaspoon garlic powder
1/3 cup chicken stock (see recipe)
1/4 cup rice milk (more or less as needed for desired consistency)

Start caramelizing the onions, or defrost if pre-made in freezer. While onions are cooking or thawing out, pierce potatoes with fork and arrange on paper towels in microwave oven. Microwave on high 10 minutes or until done, turning potatoes after 5 minutes. Remove and let stand 5 minutes. Cut each potato in half lengthwise and scoop out pulp, leaving a 1/4-inch shell. Combine potato pulp with oil, salt, pepper, garlic powder and chicken stock. Mash well. Add rice milk a little at a time and continue to mash until desired consistency is reached. You want the potatoes to be fluffy but still retain their shape. Spoon mashed potato mixture evenly back into shells. Set aside at room temperature until caramelized onions are done. When ready to serve, arrange potatoes on a microwave-safe plate and microwave for 30 seconds. Top evenly with hot caramelized onion mixture and serve. Makes 6 servings.

Cauliflower with Capers, Raisins and Breadcrumbs

1 large head cauliflower, cut into flowerets
6 tablespoons extra virgin olive oil, divided
Sea salt and freshly ground black pepper
4 garlic cloves, thinly sliced
2 tablespoons capers, drained
3/4 cup breadcrumbs (see bread recipes)
1/2 cup chicken stock (see recipe)
1/3 cup golden raisins
1 tablespoon white wine vinegar
3 tablespoons fresh parsley, chopped

Preheat oven to 425°F. Place cauliflower flowerets and 3 tablespoons oil in large bowl and toss well to coat. Season with salt and pepper. Spread mixture in a single layer on large rimmed baking sheet. Roast, tossing occasionally, until golden and crispy, about 45 minutes. Heat remaining oil over medium-low heat in small saucepan. Add garlic and cook, stirring occasionally, until slightly golden, about 5 to 6 minutes. Add capers and cook until they start to pop, about 3 minutes. Add breadcrumbs and mix well to coat. Cook, stirring constantly, until breadcrumbs begin to turn golden, about 2 to 3 minutes. Transfer breadcrumb mixture to plate and set aside. Add chicken stock to same saucepan and bring to boil. Add raisins and vinegar. Bring to boil, then reduce heat to medium-low and simmer until almost all liquid is absorbed, about 5 minutes. Remove from heat and set aside. Transfer warm cauliflower to a large serving bowl. Scatter raisin mixture over top, then toss to mix well. Season to taste with salt and pepper. Just before serving, sprinkle breadcrumb mixture and parsley over top, and toss well. Serve immediately. Makes 8 to 10 servings.

Honey Roasted Squash

2-1/2 pounds winter squash
1/4 cup corn-free honey (see note)
3 tablespoons extra-virgin olive oil
1/4 teaspoon sea salt
1 teaspoon cinnamon
Pinch of nutmeg

Preheat oven to 450°F. Cut squash in half and remove guts. Cut into quarters and arrange skin side down on rimmed, foil lined baking sheet. Drizzle with 2 tablespoons oil then toss to coat all pieces. Sprinkle with salt. Roast 10 minutes. In small saucepan over medium-high heat, whisk honey with 1 tablespoon oil, cinnamon and pinch of nutmeg and bring to simmer. Brush over squash and drizzle any remaining mixture over top. Roast until tender, basting every 10 minutes, roughly 30 to 35 minutes total. Place squash on a serving dish and drizzle evenly with juices. Makes 4 servings.

Always use caution when buying honey. Unless you buy certified 100% pure organic, it may contain unlabeled high fructose corn syrup. Honey can be replaced with agave nectar in many recipes.

Mashed Potatoes

2 pounds russet potatoes, peeled and chopped
1/2 cup chicken stock (see recipe)
1/2 cup rice milk
1 tablespoons extra-virgin olive oil
1/4 teaspoon garlic powder
Sea salt and freshly ground white pepper to taste

Bring a large saucepan of water to a full boil over high heat. Add potatoes. Reduce heat, cover and simmer until potatoes are tender, 20 to 25 minutes. In small bowl, mix stock and rice milk together. Drain potatoes and oil, then add stock rice milk mixture a little at a time, mashing as you go, until the desired consistency is reached. Add garlic powder, and salt and pepper. Mash into potatoes. Serve hot. Makes 6 to 8 servings.

Mixed Vegetable Curry

3 tablespoons extra-virgin olive oil
1 onion, sliced
1 teaspoon ground cumin
1 teaspoon chili powder
2 teaspoons ground coriander
1 teaspoon ground turmeric
2 medium sized potatoes, diced
1-1/2 cups cauliflower flowerets
3/4 cup green beans, sliced
1 cup carrots, diced
4 tomatoes, peeled and chopped
1-1/4 cups hot vegetable stock (see recipe)

Heat oil over medium-high heat in large skillet. Add onion and cook until softened, about 5 minutes. Stir in cumin, chili powder, coriander and turmeric and cook for 2 minutes. Add potatoes, cauliflower, green beans and carrots. Mix well with spices until coated. Add tomatoes and stock and cover. Bring to a boil then reduce heat and simmer 10 to 12 minutes, or until vegetable are tender. Serve hot. Makes 4 servings.

Mushrooms with Potatoes and Herbs

2 tablespoons fresh parsley, finely chopped
2 tablespoons fresh marjoram, finely chopped
1/3 cup extra-virgin olive oil
4 cloves garlic, minced
1 pound potatoes, peeled and chopped into small chunks
1 pound wild mushrooms, trimmed and thinly sliced
12 ounces button mushrooms, thinly sliced
Sea salt and freshly ground black pepper to taste

Heat 3 tablespoons oil over medium heat in large skillet. If using fresh parsley and marjoram, add to pan and sauté 1 minute. If using dry, add with potatoes and sauté until potatoes are almost tender, 5 to 10 minutes. Transfer potatoes to bowl and set aside. Heat remaining oil over medium-high heat in same skillet. Add mushrooms and sear until golden brown, 5 to 7 minutes. If a liquid develops, tilt skillet and remove with a spoon or paper towel. Just as mushrooms start to brown, reduce heat to medium, add garlic and sauté until fragrant, 1 to 2 minutes. Add potatoes back into skillet and sauté until hot, 2 to 3 minutes. Season with salt and pepper to taste. Serve hot. Makes 4 to 6 servings.

Okra and Tomatoes Masala

1 pound okra, sliced in 3/4 inch pieces
4 Roma tomatoes, diced
1 yellow onion, diced
2 green chilies
1 tablespoon Garam Masala (see recipe)
1/2 teaspoon garlic, minced
1/2 teaspoon fresh ginger, grated
1 teaspoon red chili powder
3 tablespoons extra-virgin olive oil
1/2 bunch cilantro, finely chopped
Sea salt to taste
1 bay leaf
1/8 teaspoon onion powder

Heat oil over medium-high heat in heavy skillet. Add onions, bay leaf and garlic powder and sauté until onions are tender and light brown. Add chilies, ginger and garlic and sauté 1 minute. Add 1/2 tablespoon Garam Masala and sauté 2 minutes. Mix in okra, tomatoes, red chili powder and salt. Cover and cook until tomatoes become soft, 3 to 4 minutes. Make sure okra does not stick to skillet. Cook 2 more minutes, then remove skillet from heat. Sprinkle another 1/2 tablespoon Garam Masala on top. Garnish with cilantro and serve hot. Makes 2 to 4 servings.

Roasted Beets

6 large beets
2 small yellow onions, trimmed and outer skin peeled off
2 tablespoons balsamic vinegar
2 tablespoons extra-virgin olive oil
2 cloves garlic, minced
Sea salt and freshly ground black pepper to taste
1 tablespoon fresh parsley, chopped (optional)

Preheat oven to 400°F. Wash beets and place in a baking dish just big enough to hold beets and onions without crowding them. Cover and roast about 55 minutes, stirring occasionally, until you can stick a sharp knife into center of the beets fairly easily. Remove from oven. In small bowl, mix vinegar, olive oil and garlic. When beets and onions have cooled enough to handle, peel and cut into bite-sized pieces. Toss with vinegar mixture. Add salt and pepper to taste. Top with chopped parsley, if desired. Makes 4 servings.

Roasted Potatoes

4 tablespoons extra-virgin olive oil
4 large Idaho potatoes, peeled and cut into 1/8-inch slices
20 fresh or dried bay leaves
Coarsely ground sea salt to taste

Preheat oven to 450°F. Grease a large, rimmed baking sheet with 1/2 tablespoon oil. Spread potato slices out in long rows in prepared baking sheet. Insert bay leaves between potato slices at even intervals. Drizzle with remaining olive oil, and season with salt. Roast potatoes, turning the pan halfway through cooking, until the edges are crisp and the centers are tender, about 1 hour. Season with more salt to taste. Serve hot or at room temperature. Makes 8 servings.

Roasted Red Peppers

6 to 8 large red peppers, cored, seeded, and chopped into large
    chunks
3 cloves garlic, minced
1/2 cup tightly packed fresh basil leaves
2 tablespoons extra-virgin olive oil

Preheat oven to 425°F. Place peppers, garlic and basil in large bowl.
Add oil and mix well to coat. Using a slotted spoon, scoop mixture
onto wide roasting pan. Roast at least 1 hour, stirring every 20
minutes. When peppers are soft and beginning to blacken on the
corners, remove from heat and allow to set for at least 1 hour.
Freezes well. Makes 3 to 4 cups.

Roasted Vegetables

1 eggplant, cut into 1-inch cubes
1 large or 2 small zucchini, cut into 1-inch cubes
1 red pepper, cored, seeded, and chopped into 1-inch pieces
5 small squash, thickly sliced
Large handful of fresh green beans, trimmed
1 red onion, cut into wedges
1/2 cup fresh basil leaves, packed
1 sprig of fresh rosemary
1 tablespoon fresh thyme leaves, removed from stems
2 tablespoons extra-virgin olive oil
3 large ripe tomatoes, roughly chopped
3 cloves garlic, minced

Preheat oven to 450°F. Place zucchini and eggplant in colander in
sink and salt them evenly. Allow to drain for 30 minutes. Pat dry
before adding to roasting pan. Place pepper, squash, beans, onion,
herbs, tomatoes, and garlic into roasting pan. Drizzle oil over pan
and toss to coat evenly. Roast for approximately 1 to 1-1/2 hours,
stirring every 15 minutes, until vegetables are tender and deeply
browned. Leftovers can be frozen for later use to flavor or thicken
soups and stews. Makes 6 to 8 servings.

Sausage Stuffed Mushrooms

24 large stuffing mushrooms, stems removed and reserved
3 tablespoons extra-virgin olive oil, divided
3 cloves garlic, minced
1 package Al Fresco Fresh Sweet Italian Style Chicken Sausages,
    skinned
1/2 medium white onion, grated
3/4 cup bread crumbs (see bread recipes)
1-1/2 tablespoons fresh parsley, chopped
1/2 teaspoon sea salt

Preheat oven to 400°F. Lightly coat mushroom caps with 1
tablespoon oil. Place oiled caps in a single layer in baking dish.
Chop half of reserved mushroom stems and set aside. Discard
remaining stems or save for another use. Heat remaining 2
tablespoons of oil in large skillet over medium-high heat. Add garlic
and sauté until fragrant, about 2 minutes. Add sausage and cook
until browned, stirring frequently. Break up bigger pieces as it
cooks. Add pepper, onion, and chopped mushroom stems.
Continue to cook until vegetables are tender, about 3 to 5 minutes.
Remove from heat and stir in bread crumbs, parsley and salt. Stir
until thoroughly combined. Fill mushroom caps with stuffing. Bake
in center of oven about 15 minutes, or until heated through. Serve
hot. Makes 8 servings.

Sautéed Green Beans

2 teaspoons plus 2 teaspoons extra-virgin olive oil
1 pound green beans, trimmed and cut into 2-inch pieces
1/4 teaspoon sea salt (more to season)
Freshly ground black pepper
3 cloves garlic, minced
1/4 cup water
1 teaspoon lemon juice
1 tablespoon fresh basil

Heat 2 teaspoons oil over medium-high heat in large skillet until it begins to smoke. Add green beans and salt and sauté until brown spots appear, 4 to 6 minutes. Move green beans aside and add rest of oil and garlic. Cook, mashing the mixture into the pan until fragrant, about 1 minute. Stir into green beans. Add water, cover and cook until bright green and still crisp, about 2 minutes. Uncover, turn heat to high and cook, stirring frequently, until water evaporates and beans are crisp-tender and lightly browned, 3 to 5 minutes. Remove from heat. Stir in lemon juice and fresh basil. Season with salt and pepper to taste. Serve hot. Makes 4 servings.

Tomatoes with Garlic, Rosemary and Olives

3 tablespoons extra-virgin olive oil
3 cloves minced garlic
2 pints cherry or grape tomatoes
10 black brined olives, pitted and sliced (see note)
1 tablespoon fresh rosemary, stemmed and chopped
1 teaspoon sea salt
1/4 teaspoon freshly ground black pepper

Heat oil over medium heat in a large skillet. Add garlic and cook 1 minute, stirring constantly. Add tomatoes, olives, rosemary, salt, and pepper. Reduce heat and simmer 5 to 7 minutes, stirring occasionally, until tomatoes start to lose their shape. Transfer to serving dish and serve hot or room temperature. Makes 6 servings. Note: Make sure the olives are brined with white wine vinegar, not distilled white vinegar, which may contain corn or gluten.

Yams with Apple Butter and Cinnamon

2 pounds yams or (can substitute sweet potatoes)
1/4 cup additive-free apple butter, more or less as desired (see
    recipe)
Pinch of sea salt
Ground cinnamon (to sprinkle on top)

Optional:
Small handful plump golden raisins
Honey, drizzle for top (see note)

Preheat the oven to 350°F. Pierce yams with fork and place on
rimmed baking sheet. Bake for 1-1/2 hours, or until tender. Peel
yams and transfer to large bowl. Add apple butter and salt, and
mash until creamy. Add more apple butter as desired for
consistency. Transfer to serving dish. Lightly sprinkle top with
cinnamon, or if you prefer, drizzle with honey, and serve hot.
Makes 5 servings.

Always use caution when buying honey. Unless you buy certified
100% pure organic, it may contain unlabeled high fructose corn
syrup. Honey can be replaced with agave nectar in many recipes.

Metric Cooking Conversions

Metric to U.S.

Capacity
    1 milliliter = 1/5 teaspoon
    5 ml = 1 teaspoon
    15 ml = 1 tablespoon
    34 ml = 1 fluid oz.
    100 ml = 3.4 fluid oz.
    240 ml = 1 cup
    1 liter = 34 fluid oz.
    1 liter = 4.2 cups
    1 liter = 2.1 pints
    1 liter = 1.06 quarts
    1 liter = .26 gallon

Weight
    1 gram = .035 ounce
    100 grams = 3.5 ounces
    500 grams = 1.10 pounds
    1 kilogram = 2.205 pounds
    1 kilogram = 35 oz.

U.S. to Metric

Capacity
    1/5 teaspoon = 1 milliliter
    1 teaspoon = 5 ml
    1 tablespoon = 15 ml
    1/5 cup = 50 ml
    1 cup = 240 ml
    2 cups (1 pint) = 470 ml
    4 cups (1 quart) = .95 liter
    4 quarts (1 gal.) = 3.8 liters

Weight
    1 fluid oz. = 30 milliliters
    1 fluid oz. = 28 grams
    1 pound = 454 grams

Oven Temperature Conversions

Fahrenheit	Celsius	Gas	
250	120	1	very slow
300	150	2	slow
325	160	3	moderately slow
350	180	4	moderate
375	190	5	moderately hot
400	200	6	hot
450	230	7	very hot
500	250	9	very hot

Cooking Measurement Equivalents

Dry Cooking Measurement Equivalents

16 tablespoons = 1 cup
12 tablespoons = 3/4 cup
10 tablespoons + 2 teaspoons = 2/3 cup
8 tablespoons = 1/2 cup
6 tablespoons = 3/8 cup
5 tablespoons + 1 teaspoon = 1/3 cup
4 tablespoons = 1/4 cup
2 tablespoons = 1/8 cup
2 tablespoons + 2 teaspoons = 1/6 cup
1 tablespoon = 1/16 cup
2 cups = 1 pint
2 pints = 1 quart
3 teaspoons = 1 tablespoon
48 teaspoons = 1 cup

Dry measure pints and quarts are not interchangeable with liquid measure pints and quarts. Dry measure is about 1/6 larger than liquid measure and is used for raw fruits and vegetables when dealing with large quantities.

Liquid Cooking Measurement Equivalents

60 drops = Less than 1/8 teaspoon
1 teaspoon = 1/3 tablespoon
1 tablespoon = 3 teaspoons
2 tablespoons = 1 fluid ounce
4 tablespoons = 1/4 cup or 2 ounces
5-1/3 tablespoons = 1/3 cup or 2-2/3 ounces
8 tablespoons = 1/2 cup or 4 ounces
16 tablespoons = 1 cup or 8 ounces or 2 gills
1/4 cup = 4 tablespoons
3/8 cup = 1/4 cup + 2 tablespoons
5/8 cup = 1/2 cup + 2 tablespoons
7/8 cup = 3/4 cup + 2 tablespoons
1 cup = 1/2 pint or 8 fluid ounces
2 cups = 1 pint or 16 fluid ounces
1 gill = 1/2 cup or 4 fluid ounces
1 pint = 4 gills or 16 fluid ounces
1 quart = 2 pints or 4 cups
1 gallon = 4 quarts

ෆ○ය

When measuring dry or solid ingredients, dip the cup or spoon measure into the food and lift out. Use the edge of a knife to scrape across the surface, removing excess ingredients so the surface is flat. When measuring liquids, place cup on flat surface bend down to check at eye level.

ෆ ය

Suggested Products

Even though the ingredients for these products have been verified on the dates listed below, always double-check with the manufacturer before buying to make sure nothing has changed.

Al Fresco Fresh Sweet Italian Style Chicken Sausages: Skinless chicken meat, red and green Bell peppers, and contains 2% or less of salt, sugar, spices (including fennel and black pepper), natural flavors (pepper, fennel, basil, red cayenne pepper, crushed red pepper, paprika, rosemary and capsicum extract) in natural pork casing. Confirmed May 8, 2012. Toll-free number: 1-800-426-6100.

Coconut Aminos: Certified organic raw coconut sap (from the blossom) and sea salt. Bottled in a facility that does not handle or process tree nuts of any kind. Toll-free number: 1-888-369-3393. Confirmed May 21, 2012.

Enjoy Life Mini-Chocolate Chips: Evaporated cane juice, chocolate liquor, non-dairy cocoa butter. Made in a dedicated nut and gluten-free facility. Toll-free number: 1-888-503-6569. Confirmed May 21, 2012.

Red Star Active Dry Yeast: 1/4-ounce packets are grown on corn-free molasses. Use caution when buying; the larger sizes contain corn in the form of an emulsifier called sorbitan monostearate. Confirmed May 8, 2012. Toll-free number: 1-800-558-7279.

Soy Free Vegenaise by Follow Your Heart. Expeller-pressed hi-oleic safflower oil, filtered water, brown rice syrup, apple cider vinegar, pea protein, sea salt, mustard flour, lemon juice concentrate. Phone: 1-818-348-3240. Confirmed May 21, 2012. Caution: Although the pea protein is not hydrolyzed, it may still contain enough naturally occurring free glutamate to serve as an MSG-trigger in highly sensitive people.

Spectrum Palm Oil Shortening: 100% organic expeller pressed palm oil. Toll-free number: 1-800-434-4246. Confirmed May 21, 2012.

Udi's au Natural Granola: Thick cut rolled oats, corn-free wildflower honey, and canola oil. Confirmed May 8, 2012. Phone: 1-303-657-6366.

Index

Lightning Source UK Ltd.
Milton Keynes UK
UKOW04f1809200214

226860UK00001B/62/P